Third Edition

Study Guide for Essentials of Nursing Research

Methods, Appraisal, and Utilization

Denise F. Polit, PhD

Humanalysis, Inc.
Saratoga Springs, New York
Formerly of the Boston College School of Nursing
Chestnut Hill, Massachusetts

Bernadette P. Hungler, RN, PhD

Boston College School of Nursing
Chestnut Hill, Massachusetts

J. B. Lippincott Company
Philadelphia

Third Edition

Study Guide for Essentials of Nursing Research

Methods, Appraisal, and Utilization

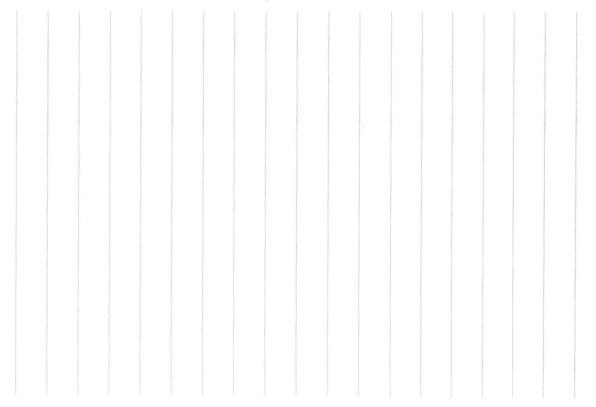

Sponsoring Editor: David P. Carroll
Manuscript Editor: Jody DeMatteo
Coordinating Editorial Assistant: Patty L. Shear
Project Editor: Mary Kinsella
Design Coordinator: Kathy Kelley-Luedtke
Production Manager: Helen Ewan
Production Coordinator: Nannette Winski
Compositor: Compset, Inc.
Printer/Binder: RR Donnelley & Sons Company

ISBN 0-397-54923-7

6 5 4 3 2 1

Preface

This study guide has been prepared to complement *Essentials of Nursing Research: Methods, Appraisal, and Utilization*. The guide provides opportunities to reinforce the acquisition of basic research skills through systematic learning exercises. The book is also intended to help bridge the gap between the passive reading of complex, abstract materials and the development of skills needed to evaluate research through concrete examples and study suggestions.

As in the case of the textbook, this study guide was developed on the premise that research examples are a critical component of the learning process. The inclusion of actual and fictitious research examples is designed to instruct (*i.e.,* facilitate the absorption of research concepts); motivate (*i.e.,* encourage students to envision the merit of acquiring research skills); and stimulate (*i.e.,* suggest topics that might be pursued further by nurse researchers and practicing nurses interested in the utilization of research findings).

This study guide consists of 14 chapters—one chapter corresponding to every chapter of the text. Each of the 14 chapters consists of five sections:

- *Matching Exercises.* Terms and concepts presented in the text are reinforced by having students perform a matching routine that often involves matching the concrete (*e.g.,* actual hypotheses) with the abstract (*e.g.,* types of hypotheses).
- *Completion Exercises.* Sentences are presented in which the student must fill in a missing word or phrase corresponding to important ideas presented in the text.
- *Study Questions.* Each chapter contains two to five short individual exercises relevant to the text materials, including the preparation of definition of terms.
- *Application Exercises.* These exercises are geared specifically to the consumers of nursing research and involve opportunities to critique various aspects of a study. Each chapter contains both fictitious research examples and suggestions for actual research reports, which students are asked to evaluate according to a dimension emphasized in the corresponding chapter of the text. A new feature of this edition is the inclusion of two complete studies for students' critical appraisal.
- *Special Projects.* This section offers suggestions for fairly large projects in which, in many cases, an entire classroom could collaborate.

Contents

Study Guide for Essentials of Nursing Research

Methods, Appraisal, and Utilization

Introduction to Nursing Research

Part I

‖‖‖‖ Chapter 1
Fundamentals of
Nursing Research

‖ A. MATCHING EXERCISES

1. Match each of the activities in Set B with one of the time frames in Set A. Indicate the letter corresponding to the appropriate response next to each entry in Set B.

Set A

a. Pre-1950s
b. 1950s and 1960s
c. 1970s to present
d. None of the above

Set B   *Responses*

1. Nursing research focused on nurses themselves   _____
2. Increased research focus on clinical problems   _____
3. Establishment of the National Center for Nursing Research at the National Institutes of Health   _____
4. Creation of the professional journal *Research in Nursing and Health*   _____
5. First nursing research study was conducted   _____
6. Creation of the professional journal *Nursing Research*   _____
7. Increased interest in theoretical bases for conducting nursing research   _____
8. Federal funding becomes available to support nursing research   _____
9. Growing interest of nurse researchers in conducting in-depth, process-oriented studies   _____
10. Two professional nursing research journals cease publication due to low circulation   _____

▌ B. COMPLETION EXERCISES

Write the words or phrases that correctly complete the sentences below.

1. Research in nursing began with _____.
2. During the early years, most nursing studies focused on _____
   _____.
3. The rapid acceleration of nursing research began in the _____
   _____.
4. The future direction of nursing research is likely to involve a continuing focus
   on _____.
5. The most ingrained source of knowledge, and the one that is the most difficult
   to challenge, is _____.
6. The approach to human knowledge that uses systematic, controlled procedures
   is known as the _____.
7. The scientific assumption that all phenomena have antecedent causes is called
   _____.
8. Evidence that is rooted in objective reality and gathered through the human
   senses is known as _____.
9. Since scientific inquiry is not concerned with isolated phenomena, a key characteristic of the scientific method is _____.
10. Of the various purposes of scientific inquiry, the one that epitomizes its spirit is
    _____.
11. The scientific approach has as its philosophical underpinnings a school of
    thought known as _____.
12. The philosophical perspective that has challenged the traditional scientific ap-
    proach on the grounds that it is overly reductionist is known as the _____
    _____ perspective.

▌ C. STUDY QUESTIONS

1. Define the following terms. Use the textbook to compare your definition with
   the definition in Chapter 1 or in the Glossary.
   a. Producer of nursing research: _____
   _____
   _____
   b. Consumer of nursing research: _____
   _____
   _____

  c. National Center for Nursing Research: _____

  _____

  _____

  d. Scientific method: _____

  _____

  _____

  e. Assumption: _____

  _____

  _____

  f. Applied research: _____

  _____

  _____

  g. Basic research: _____

  _____

  _____

  h. Qualitative research: _____

  _____

  _____

  i. Quantitative research: _____

  _____

  _____

2. Why is it important for nurses who will never conduct their own research to understand scientific methods?

3. What are some potential consequences to the profession of nursing if nurses stopped conducting their own research?

4. Many students have concerns about courses on research methods. Complete the following sentences, expressing as honestly as possible your own feelings about research, and discuss your concerns with your class.

a. I (am/am not) looking forward to this class on nursing research because:

_____

_____

b. I think that I would like a course in nursing research methods better if:

_____

_____

c. I think a class in nursing research (will/will not) improve my effectiveness as a nurse because:

_____

_____

5. Explain the ways in which scientific knowledge differs from knowledge based on tradition, authority, trial and error, and logical reasoning.

6. How does the assumption of scientific determinism conflict with or coincide with superstitious thinking? Take, as an example, the superstition associated with a four-leaf clover or a rabbit's foot.

7. Below are several research problems. For each, indicate whether you think it is *primarily* an applied or basic research question.

Research Problem	*Type*
a. Does movement tempo affect perception of the passage of time?	_____
b. Does follow-up by nurses improve patients' compliance with their medication regimens?	_____
c. Does the ingestion of cranberry juice reduce urinary tract infections?	_____
d. Is sweat gland activity related to ACTH levels?	_____

e. Is pain perception associated with a person's locus of control
(an aspect of personality)?   _____

f. Does the type of nursing curriculum affect attrition rates in
schools of nursing?   _____

g. Does nicotine affect postural muscle tremor?   _____

h. Does the nurse/patient ratio affect nurses' job satisfaction?   _____

8. Below are descriptions of several research problems. Indicate whether you think
the problem is best suited to a qualitative or quantitative approach, and indicate
why you think this is so.

    a. What is the decision-making process of AIDS patients seeking treatment?

    b. What effect does room temperature have on the colonization rate of bacteria
in urinary catheters?

    c. What are the sources of stress among nursing home residents?

    d. Does therapeutic touch affect the vital signs of hospitalized patients?

9. What are some of the limitations of quantitative research? What are some of the
limitations of qualitative research? Which approach seems best suited to address
problems in which you might be interested? Why is that?

▌ D. APPLICATION EXERCISES

1. Stewart (1993)* studied the effect of the wording of communications on encouraging the elderly to come forward for a flu vaccination. All members of a senior citizens center in a mid-sized community (a total of 500 elderly men and women) were sent a letter advising them that a flu epidemic was anticipated that season and that the elderly were especially likely to benefit from an immunization. Half of the members were sent a letter stressing the benefits of getting a flu shot. The other half of the members were sent a letter stressing the potential dangers of *not* getting a flu shot. To avoid any biases, a lottery-type system was used to determine who got which letter. All the elderly were advised that free immunizations would be available at a community health clinic over a 1-week period and that free transportation would also be made available to them. Stewart monitored the rates of coming forward for a flu shot among the two groups of elderly to assess whether one approach of encouragement was more persuasive than the other.

Consider the aspects of this study in relation to the issues discussed in this chapter. To assist you in your review, here are some guiding questions.

   a. Discuss the relevance of this study to nursing. Does it address a priority area discussed in Box 1-1 of the textbook?
   b. Do the features of this study correspond to the characteristics of the scientific approach? To what extent are the characteristics of order, control, empiricism, generalization, and theory represented in this example?
   c. How would you characterize the purpose of this study? Is its major aim description, exploration, explanation, prediction, or control? Is there more than one purpose? Would you say this study is an example of basic or applied research?
   d. Review the various limitations of the scientific method discussed in Chapter 1 and consider whether and how each applies to the study under consideration.
   e. In this study, would it be more appropriate to collect and analyze qualitative or quantitative information? Why do you think this is so?

2. Below are several suggested research articles. Skim one or more of these articles and respond to parts **a** to **e** of Question D.1 in terms of an actual research study:

   ■ Kilpack, V., Boehm, J., Smith, N., & Mudge, B. (1991). Using research-based interventions to decrease patient falls. *Applied Nursing Research, 4,* 50–56.
   ■ Mattson, S. (1990). Coping and developmental maturity of R.N. baccalaureate students. *Western Journal of Nursing Research, 12,* 514–524.

---

*This example is fictitious.

- Norman, E., Gadaleta, D., & Griffin, C. C. (1991). An evaluation of three blood pressure methods in a stabilized acute trauma population. *Nursing Research, 40,* 86–89.
- Stainton, M. C. (1992). Mismatched caring in high-risk perinatal situations. *Clinical Nursing Research, 1,* 35–49.

‖ E. SPECIAL PROJECTS

1. Consider the following research statement:

> *The purpose of this study is to determine whether patients in intensive care units are or are not satisfied with their nursing care.*

The basic purpose of this study as stated is descriptive. Alter the statement in such a way as to design a study whose essential purpose is exploration; explanation; prediction; and control.

2. Think of the last fact you learned with respect to clinical nursing practice. Try to discover the ultimate source of this information. Was it tradition ("this is the way it's always been done"); authorities ("Dr. So-and-so said so"); logical reasoning ("this has been inferred from previous observations"); or scientific method ("an empirical investigation discovered this to be the case")?

Chapter 2

Overview of the Research Process

|| A. MATCHING EXERCISES

1. Match each of the terms in Set B with one (or more) of the terms in Set A. Indicate the letter corresponding to your response next to each item in Set B.

Set A

a. Categorical variable
b. Continuous variable
c. Constant

Set B   *Responses*

1. Employment status (working/not working)   _____
2. Dosage of a new drug   _____
3. Pi (π) (to calculate area of a circle)   _____
4. Number of times hospitalized   _____
5. Method of teaching patients (structured versus unstructured)   _____
6. Blood type   _____
7. pH level of urine   _____
8. Pulse rate of a deceased person   _____
9. Membership (versus nonmembership) in a nursing
   organization   _____
10. Birth weight of an infant   _____
11. Presence or absence of decubitus   _____
12. Degree of empathy in nurses   _____

2. Match each of the terms in Set B with one of the terms in Set A. Indicate the letter corresponding to your response next to each item in Set B.

Set A

a. Independent variable
b. Dependent variable
c. Either/both

Set B   *Response*

1. The variable that is the presumed effect   _____
2. The variable that is categorical   _____
3. The variable that is the main outcome of interest in the study   _____
4. The variable that is the presumed cause   _____
5. The variable referred to as the criterion variable   _____
6. The variable that is an attribute   _____
7. The variable, "length of stay in hospital"   _____
8. The variable that requires an operational definition   _____

▌ B. COMPLETION EXERCISES

Write the words or phrases that correctly complete the sentences below.

1. The person who is the leader of a team of researchers is known as the _____ _____ or _____ .

2. The people who are being studied in a research project are often referred to as the _____ .

3. The abstract qualities in which a researcher is interested are referred to in scientific parlance as _____ or _____ _____ .

4. The variable that the researcher wants to understand, explain, or predict is known as the _____ or _____ _____variable.

5. The variable presumed to *cause* changes in some other variable is the _____ _____ .

6. If a researcher studied the effect of a scheduling assignment on nurses' morale, scheduling assignment would be referred to as the _____ variable.

7. A variable that is irrelevant in an investigation and needs to be controlled is called a(n) _____ .

8. The pieces of information obtained in the course of a study are collectively known as the _____ .

9. When a researcher carefully specifies the steps that must be taken to measure the concepts of interest, the researcher develops _____ .

10. The researcher's expectations about how variables under investigation are related are stated in the _____ .

11. The overall plan for collecting and analyzing scientific data is called the _____ .

12. Research in which the investigator plays an active, interventive role is called _____ research.

13. The total aggregate of units that a researcher is interested in is known as the _____ .

14. The actual group of study participants selected from a larger group is known as the _____ .

15. The primary criterion by which a sample is assessed for adequacy is its _____ of the population.

16. The plan for transforming research information into a numeric format suitable for analysis is called _____ .

17. A small-scale trial run of a research study is referred to as a(n) _____ .

18. Typically, the most time-consuming phase of the study is the _____ phase.

19. The task of organizing the information collected in a study is known as _____ .

20. The final phase of a research project is known as the _____ phase.

▌ C. STUDY QUESTIONS

1. Define the following terms. Use the textbook to compare your definition with the definition in Chapter 2 or in the Glossary.

   a. Investigator: _____

   _____

   _____

   b. Construct: _____

   _____

   _____

   c. Operational definition: _____

   _____

   _____

   d. Variable: _____

   _____

   _____

e. Constant: _____

_____

_____

f. Heterogeneity: _____

_____

_____

g. Relationship: _____

_____

_____

h. Cause-and-effect relationship: _____

_____

_____

i. Functional relationship: _____

_____

_____

j. Control: _____

_____

_____

2. Suggest operational definitions for the following concepts.

a. Stress: _____

_____

_____

b. Prematurity of infants: _____

_____

_____

c. Nursing effectiveness: _____

_____

_____

d. Prolonged labor: _____

_____

_____

e. Nurses' job satisfaction: _____

_____

_____

f. Respiratory function: _____

_____

_____

3. In each of the following research problems, identify the independent variables and dependent variables.

a. Does assertiveness training improve the effectiveness of psychiatric nurses?

Independent: _____

Dependent: _____

b. Does the postural positioning of patients affect their respiratory function?

Independent: _____

Dependent: _____

c. Is the psychological well-being of patients affected by the amount of touch received from nursing staff?

Independent: _____

Dependent: _____

d. Is the incidence of decubitus reduced by more frequent turnings of patients?

Independent: _____

Dependent: _____

e. Is the educational preparation of nurses related to their subsequent turnover rate?

Independent: _____

Dependent: _____

f. Is tolerance for pain related to a patient's age and gender?

Independent: _____

Dependent: _____

g. Are the number of prenatal visits of pregnant women associated with labor and delivery outcomes?

Independent: _____

Dependent: _____

h. Are levels of stress among nurses higher in pediatric or adult intensive care units?

Independent: _____

Dependent: _____

i. Are student nurses' clinical grades related to their subsequent on-the-job performances?

Independent: _____

Dependent: _____

j. Is anxiety in surgical patients affected by structured preoperative teaching?

Independent: _____

Dependent: _____

k. Are nurses' promotions related to their level of participation in continuing education activities?

Independent: _____

Dependent: _____

l. Does hearing acuity of the elderly change as a function of the time of day?

Independent: _____

Dependent: _____

m. Is patient satisfaction with nursing care related to the congruity of nurses' and patients' cultural backgrounds?

Independent: _____

Dependent: _____

n. Is a woman's educational background related to breast self-examination practices?

Independent: _____

Dependent: _____

o. Does home birth affect the parents' satisfaction with the childbirth experience?

Independent: _____

Dependent: _____

4. For each of the variables in Question C.3, indicate which is a categorical variable and which is a continuous variable.

‖ D. APPLICATION EXERCISES

1. Hebert (1993)* observed that different patients react differently to sensory overload in the hospital. She conducted a study to see whether the patients' home environments affect their reactions to hospital noises. Below are the investigator's operational definitions of the research variables.

Independent Variable: Type of home environment. Based on the patients' self-reports at intake, home environment was defined as the number of household members residing with the patient.

———————

*This example is fictitious.

Dependent Variable: Reaction to hospital noise. Based on responses to five questions answered at discharge, patients were classified as "dissatisfied with noise level" or "not dissatisfied with noise level."

Extraneous Variables:
- Age: calculated to the nearest year based on information regarding date of birth reported at intake
- Sex: patient's gender as recorded on intake form
- Social class: patient's occupation as recorded on intake form

Review and comment on these specifications. Suggest alternatives and compare the adequacy and completeness of your suggestions with the descriptions provided above. To aid you in this task, here are some guiding questions.

a. Are the operational definitions sufficiently detailed? Do they tell the reader exactly how each variable is to be measured? Can you expand any of the definitions so that they are more precise?

b. Are the operational definitions good definitions—that is, is there a better way to measure, say, home environment?

c. Has the researcher identified reasonable extraneous variables—that is, are these extraneous variables likely to be related to both the dependent variables and the independent variables?

d. Are there extraneous variables that the researcher failed to identify but that should be controlled? Suggest two or three additional extraneous variables.

2. Below are several suggested research articles. Read one of these articles and respond to parts **a** to **d** of Question D.1 in critiquing this actual reserach study. Also use the guidelines in Box 2-1 of the textbook to do a preliminary assessment of other aspects of the study.

- Beach, E. K., Maloney, B. H., Plocica, A. R., Sherry, S. E., Weaver, M., Luthringer, L., & Utz, S. (1992). The spouse: A factor in recovery after acute myocardial infarction. *Heart and Lung, 21,* 30–38.
- Dilorio, C., Faherty, B., & Manteuffel, B. (1992). Self-efficacy and social support in self-management of epilepsy. *Western Journal of Nursing Research, 14,* 292–303.
- Heitkemper, M., Jarrett, M., Bond, E. F., & Turner, P. (1991). GI symptoms, function, and psychophysiological arousal in dysmenorrheic women. *Nursing Research, 40,* 20–26.
- Thiele, J. E., Holloway, J., Murphy, D., Pendarvis, J., & Stucky, M. (1991). Perceived and actual decision making by novice baccalaureate students. *Western Journal of Nursing Research, 13,* 616–626.
- Travis, S. S., & Moore, S. R. (1991). Nursing and medical care of primary dementia patients in a community hospital setting. *Applied Nursing Research, 4,* 14–18.

▌ E. SPECIAL PROJECTS

Below is a list of variables. For each, think of a research problem for which the variable would be the independent variable and a second for which it would be the dependent variable. For example, take the variable "birth weight of infants." We might ask, "Does the age of the mother affect the birth weight of her infant?" (dependent variable). Alternatively, we could define our research question as, "Does the birth weight of infants (independent variable) affect their sensorimotor development at 6 months of age?" HINT: For the dependent variable problem, ask yourself, "What factors might affect, influence, or cause this variable?" For the independent variable, ask yourself, "What factors might *this* variable influence, cause, or affect?"

a. Body temperature

Independent: _____

Dependent: _____

b. Amount of sleep

Independent: _____

Dependent: _____

c. Compliance with a medication regimen

Independent: _____

Dependent: _____

d. Level of hopefulness in patients

Independent: _____

Dependent: _____

e. Amount of saliva secretion

Independent: _____

Dependent: _____

‖‖‖‖ Chapter 3
Research Reports: Reading and Reviewing Scientific Literature

‖ A. MATCHING EXERCISES

1. Below, under Set B, are a number of fictitious references from the *International Nursing Index*. Identify the portion of the reference that is <u>underlined</u> and match it with a term in Set A. Indicate the letter corresponding to the appropriate response next to each entry in Set B.

Set A

a. Journal
b. Volume
c. Pages

d. Issue
e. Author
f. Title

Set B

Responses

1. Convalescence following a hysterectomy. Porras T. <u>Nurs Res</u> 1992 Mar; 41(2): 157–162 _____

2. Nursing care program for bed-confined patients. <u>Gussman G.</u> Nurs Clin North Am 1991 Jan; 26(1): 83–96 _____

3. Nurse counseling following an abortion. Sala M. J Adv Nurs 1989 Nov; 9(<u>6</u>):350–357 _____

4. Level of activation and respiratory function. Mosley M. Nurs Res 1991 Jul; 40(4): <u>196–202</u> _____

5. Holistic care in a community health center. Kamphaus M. Nurs Clin North Am 1990 Feb; <u>27</u>(2): 101–115 _____

6. Treating bacteriuria in female patients with indwelling catheters. Porcelli P. Nurs Outlook 1990 Dec; 33(12): <u>770–779</u> _____

7. <u>Services for children with diabetes.</u> Thonn S. Pediatrics 1991 Jan; 64(1): 15–20 _____

8. Screening for scoliosis in school-age children. Jefferson M. J Sch Health 1989 May; 59(<u>5</u>): 315–319 _____

▌ B. COMPLETION EXERCISES

Write the words or phrases that correctly complete the sentences below.

1. The type of research reports that students are most likely to read are _____ .

2. The oldest scholarly journal that has served as an outlet for nurses engaged in scientific research is _____ .

3. The six sections typically found in research journal articles are: _____
   _____ , _____
   _____ , _____
   _____ , and _____ .

4. The most relevant index for materials specific to nursing is the _____
   _____ .

5. When a computer search yields many references, the references are generally produced _____ .

6. The computer database most often used in literature searches by nurses is _____ .

7. The two types of information that have the least utility in a research review are _____ and _____ .

8. The most important type of information to be included in a written research review is _____ .

9. Quantity of references is less important in a good literature review than the _____ of the references.

10. The written literature review should paraphrase materials and use a minimum of _____ .

11. The literature review should make clear not only what is known about a problem but also any _____ in the research.

12. The review should conclude with a _____ .

13. The literature review should be written in a language of _____ , in keeping with the limits of existing methods.

14. No hypothesis or theory can be definitely _____ or _____ by the scientific method.

▌ C. STUDY QUESTIONS

1. Define the following terms. Use the textbook to compare your definition with the definition in Chapter 3 or in the Glossary.

a. Literature review: _____

_____

_____

b. Primary source: _____

_____

_____

c. Secondary source: _____

_____

_____

d. Key word: _____

_____

_____

e. Index: _____

_____

_____

f. Abstract: _____

_____

_____

g. On-line search: _____

_____

_____

h. End-user system: _____

_____

_____

i. Poster session: _____

_____

_____

2. Below are fictitious excerpts from literature reviews. Each excerpt has a stylistic problem for a research review. Change each sentence to make it acceptable stylistically.

Original   *Revised*

a. Most elderly people do not eat a balanced diet.

b. Patient characteristics have a significant impact on nursing workload.

c. A child's conception of appropriate sick role behavior changes as the child grows older.

d. Home birth poses many potential dangers.

e. Multiple sclerosis results in considerable anxiety to the family of the patient.

f. Studies have proved that most nurses prefer not to work the night shift.

g. Life changes are the major cause of stress in adults.

h. Stroke rehabilitation programs are most effective when they involve the patients' families.

i. It has been proved that psychiatric outpatients have higher than normal rates of accidental deaths and suicides.

j. Nursing faculty are increasingly involved in conducting their own research.

k. Sickle cell counseling has emerged as an important service in community health centers.

l. The traditional pelvic examination is sufficiently unpleasant to many women that they avoid having the examination.

m. It is known that most tonsillectomies performed two decades ago were unnecessary.

n. Few smokers seriously try to break the smoking habit.

o. Severe cutaneous burns often result in hemorrhagic gastric erosions.

3. Below are several problem statements. Indicate one or more terms or key words that you would use to begin a literature search on this topic.

Problem Statement	*Key Words*
a. How effective are nurse practitioners versus pediatricians with respect to telephone management of acute pediatric illness?	_____
b. Does contingency contracting improve patient compliance with a treatment regimen?	_____
c. Does induced abortion affect the outcome of subsequent pregnancies?	_____
d. Is the amount of money a person spends on food related to the adequacy of nutrient intake?	_____
e. Is rehabilitation after spinal cord injury affected by the age and social class of the patient?	_____
f. Does the leadership style of head nurses affect the job tension and job performance of the nursing staff?	_____
g. Is loss of appetite among cancer patients associated with reactions to chemotherapy?	_____
h. What is the effect of alcohol skin preparation before insulin injection on the incidence of local and systemic infection?	_____
i. Are bottle-fed babies introduced to solid foods sooner than breast-fed babies?	_____
j. Do children raised on vegetarian diets have different growth patterns than do other children?	_____

4. Read Susan Kelley's (1990) study entitled "Parental stress response to sexual abuse and ritualistic abuse of children in day care centers," which appeared in *Nursing Research, 39,* pages 25–29. Write a summary of the problem, methods, findings, and conclusions of the study. Your summary should be capable of serving as notes for a review of the literature on child abuse by child care providers.

‖ D. APPLICATION EXERCISES

1. Below is an excerpt from White's (1992)* literature review dealing with pelvic inflammatory disease.

> *There are no universally accepted criteria for defining pelvic inflammatory disease (PID) or for categorizing its severity. Furthermore, PID does not exhibit uniformity in its clinical features. Etiologically, cases of acute PID can be divided on the basis of those caused by Neisseria gonorrhoeae, those caused by nongonococcal bacteria, and those caused by a combination of both. Eschenbach and his colleagues (1980) have reported that approximately half of the women with PID whom they examined had gonococcal infections. Eschenbach (1984) has noted that "this difference in etiological agents may explain the clinical differences between the gonococcal and nongonococcal PID. The latter may appear less acute and may not demonstrate many of the well-defined clinical features associated with gonorrhea" (p. 148). Both gonococcal and nongonococcal PID may result in subsequent obstruction of the fallopian tubes, which is among the most common causes of infertility in women. Since fertilized eggs remain in the fallopian tubes for approximately 3 days, they must provide nourishment for the developing zygote. Thus, even a tube that is not completely blocked, but that is severely damaged, can contribute to infertility.*
>
> *Westrom (1980), in a study of women treated for PID, proved that PID has an impact on subsequent fertility. A sample of 415 women with laparoscopically confirmed PID were reviewed after 9.5 years and compared with 100 control subjects who had never been treated for PID. Among the 415 women who had had PID, 88 (21.2%) were involuntarily childless; of these 88, the failure to conceive was due to tubal obstruction in 72 cases (82%). A total of 263 of the 415 subjects (63.4%) had become pregnant. In the control group, only three women (3%) were involuntarily childless.*
>
> *Westrom's study also revealed a relationship between infertility and the number of PID infections. Tubal occlusion was diagnosed after one infection in 32 women (12.8%); after two infections in 22 cases (35.5%); and after three or more in-*

---

*This example is fictitious.

fections in 18 cases (75.5%). Of the 415 women with acute PID in Westrom's sample, 94 (22.7%) experienced more than one infection. Evidence from other studies confirms that a large percentage of women with PID have a history of previous PID and that recurrent PID usually has a nongonococcal etiology (Jacobson & Westrom, 1984; Ringrose, 1980; Eschenbach, 1981).

The number of women affected by PID annually in the United States is unknown and difficult to estimate. According to Rose (1986), Eschenbach and colleagues used data from the National Disease and Therapeutic Index Study and the Hospital Record Study to estimate that over 500,000 cases of PID occurred annually in the United States in the early 1980s. The information from the Hospital Record Study indicated that a mean of over 160,000 patients with PID were hospitalized annually from 1980 through 1983.

Critique this literature review in regard to the points made in Chapter 3 of the textbook. To assist you in this task, you can answer the guiding questions below as well as the applicable questions in Box 3-3 of the textbook.

a. Is the review well organized? Does the author skip from theme to theme in a disjointed way, or is there a logic to the order of presentation of materials?

b. Is the content of the review appropriate? Does the author use secondary sources when a primary source was available? Are all the references relevant, or does the inclusion of some material appear contrived? Do you have a sense that the author was thorough in uncovering all the relevant materials? Do the references seem outdated? Is there an overdependence on opinion articles or anecdotes? Are prior studies merely summarized, or are their shortcomings discussed? Does the author indicate what is not known as well as what is?

c. Does the style seem appropriate for a research review? Does the review seem biased or laden with subjective opinions? Is there too little paraphrasing and too much quoting? Does the author use appropriately tentative language in describing the results of earlier studies?

2. Read the literature review section in one of the articles listed below. Critique the review, applying parts **a** to **c** of Question D.1 as well as the questions in Box 3-3 of the textbook.

- Conn, V. (1991). Self-care actions taken by older adults for influenza and colds. *Nursing Research, 40,* 176–181.
- Davis, D. C., & Dearman, C. N. (1991). Coping strategies of infertile women. *Journal of Obstetric, Gynecologic, and Neonatal Nursing, 20,* 221–227.
- Kelly, C., Dumenko, L., McGregor, S. E., & McHutchion, M. E. (1992). A change in flushing protocols of central venous catheters. *Oncology Nursing Forum, 19,* 599–605.

- Lobo, M. L. (1992). Parent–infant interaction during feeding when the infant has congenital heart disease. *Journal of Pediatric Nursing, 7,* 97–105.
- Liehr, P., Todd, B., Rossi, M., & Culligan, M. (1992). Effect of venous support on edema and leg pain in patients after coronary artery bypass graft surgery. *Heart and Lung, 21,* 6–11.

▌ E. SPECIAL PROJECTS

1. Read the literature review section from a research article appearing in an issue of *Nursing Research* in the early 1980s (some possibilities are suggested below). Search the literature for more recent research on the topic of the article and update the review section. Don't forget to incorporate in your review the findings from the article itself! Here are some possible articles.
- Austin, J. K., McBride, A. B., & Davis, H. W. (1984). Parental attitude and adjustment to childhood epilepsy. *Nursing Research, 33,* 92–96.
- Choi-Lao, A. (1981). Trace anesthetic vapors in hospital operating-room environments. *Nursing Research, 30,* 156–161.
- Keane, A., Ducette, J., & Adler, D. (1985). Stress in ICU and non-ICU nurses. *Nursing Research, 34,* 231–236.
- Schraeder, B. D., & Cooper, B. M. (1983). Development and temperament in very low birth weight infants. *Nursing Research, 32,* 331–335.

2. Select one of the problem statements from Question C.3. Conduct a literature search and identify 5 to 10 relevant references. Compare your references with those of your classmates in terms of relevance, recency, and type of information provided.

3. Read one of the studies suggested in Question D.2. Write a two-page summary of the research report, translating the information into everyday (*i.e.,* nonresearch) language.

Preliminary Steps in the Research Process

Part II

‖‖‖ Chapter 4
Research Problems and Hypotheses

‖ A. MATCHING EXERCISES

1. Match each of the statements in Set B with one of the terms in Set A. Indicate the letter corresponding to the appropriate response next to each statement in Set B.

Set A

a. Research hypothesis—directional
b. Research hypothesis—nondirectional
c. Null hypothesis
d. Not a hypothesis as stated

Set B   *Responses*

1. First-born infants have higher concentrations of estrogens and progesterone in umbilical cord blood than do later-born infants. _____
2. There is no relationship between participation in prenatal classes and the health outcomes of infants. _____
3. Nursing students are increasingly interested in obtaining advanced degrees. _____
4. Nurse practitioners have more job mobility than do other registered nurses. _____
5. A person's age is related to his or her difficulty in accessing health care. _____
6. Glaucoma can be effectively screened by means of tonometry. _____
7. Increased noise levels result in increased anxiety among hospitalized patients. _____
8. Media exposure of the health hazards of smoking is unrelated to the public's smoking habits. _____
9. Patients' compliance with their medication regimens is correlated with their perceptions of the consequences of noncompliance. _____
10. The primary reason that nurses participate in continuing education programs is for professional advancement. _____

11. Baccalaureate, diploma, and associate degree nursing graduates differ with respect to technical and clinical skills acquired.   _____

12. A cancer patient's degree of hopefulness regarding the future is unrelated to his or her religiosity.   _____

13. The degree of attachment between children and their mothers is associated with the level of anxiety they experience during a hospitalization.   _____

14. The presence of homonymous hemianopia in stroke patients negatively affects their length of stay in the hospital.   _____

15. Adjustment to hemodialysis does not vary by the patient's gender.   _____

▌ B. COMPLETION EXERCISES

Write the words or phrases that correctly complete the sentences below.

1. The form of the problem statement can be either _____ _____ or _____ .

2. The four most common sources of ideas for research problems are _____ _____ , _____ , _____ , and _____ .

3. Unavailability of subjects would make a research project _____ _____ .

4. Moral or philosophical questions are inherently _____ .

5. Problem statements worded in the declarative form are often phrased as _____ .

6. Although it is desirable to have the problem statement placed early in a research report, the most typical location is at the end of the _____ _____ .

7. Research hypotheses state a predicted _____ between variables.

8. A hypothesis involves a prediction regarding at least _____ variables.

9. A hypothesis that states a prediction regarding two or more independent and two or more dependent variables is called a _____ or _____ hypothesis.

10. The type of hypothesis used in statistical testing is called the _____ or _____ hypothesis.

▌▌C. STUDY QUESTIONS

1. Define the following terms. Use the textbook to compare your definition with the definition in Chapter 4 or in the Glossary.

   a. Problem statement: _____

   _____

   _____

   b. Declarative problem statement: _____

   _____

   _____

   c. Interrogative problem statement: _____

   _____

   _____

   d. Hypothesis: _____

   _____

   _____

   e. Simple hypothesis: _____

   _____

   _____

   f. Complex hypothesis: _____

   _____

   _____

   g. Nondirectional hypothesis: _____

   _____

   _____

   h. Null hypothesis: _____

   _____

   _____

   i. Directional hypothesis: _____

   _____

   _____

2. Below is a list of general topics that could be investigated. Develop at least one problem statement for each. Assess the adequacy of your statement in terms of the problem's researchability and feasibility and the wording of the statement. HINT: Think of these concepts as potential independent or dependent variables. Ask, "What might cause or affect this variable?" and "What might be the consequences or effects of this variable?" This should lead to some ideas for a problem statement.

a. Patient comfort: _____

_____

_____

b. Psychiatric patients' readmission rates: _____

_____

_____

c. Anxiety in hospitalized children: _____

_____

_____

d. Student attrition from nursing school: _____

_____

_____

e. Attitudes toward artificial insemination: _____

_____

_____

f. Incidence of venereal disease: _____

_____

_____

g. Menstrual irregularities: _____

_____

_____

h. Requests for tubal ligation: _____

_____

_____

i. Elevated blood pressure: _____

_____

_____

j. Nurses' job satisfaction: _____

_____

_____

k. Patient cooperativeness in the recovery room: _____

_____

_____

l. Nutritional knowledge: _____

_____

_____

m. Mother–infant bonding: _____

_____

_____

3. Below is a list of researchable problem statements. Transform those stated in the interrogative form to the declarative form, and vice versa.

Original Version   *Transformed Version*

a. Can a program of nursing counseling affect sexual readjustment among women after a hysterectomy?

b. The purpose of the research is to study the relationship between nurses' unit assignments and their absentee rates.

c. What are the sequelae of an inadequately maintained sterile environment for tracheal suctioning?

d. What is the relationship between type A and type B personalities and speech patterns?

e. The purpose of the study is to investigate the effect of an AIDS education workshop on teenagers' understanding of AIDS and the HIV virus.

f. The purpose of the research is to study patients' responses to transfer from a coronary care unit.

g. What effect does the presence of the father in the delivery room have on the mother's satisfaction with the childbirth experience?

h. The purpose of the study is to examine the effect of clients' physical proximity to community health centers on health care utilization.

i. What is the long-term child-development effect of maternal heroin addiction during pregnancy?

j. The purpose of the research is to study the effect of spermicides on the physiologic development of the fetus.

4. Below are five nondirectional hypotheses. Restate each one as a directional hypothesis.

Nondirectional   *Directional*

a. Nurses' attitudes toward mental retarda-tion vary according to their clinical spe-cialty area.

b. Nurses and patients differ in terms of the relative importance they attach to having the patients' physical versus emotional needs met.

c. Type of nursing care (primary versus team) is unrelated to patient satisfaction with the care they receive.

d. The incidence of decubitus ulcers is re-lated to the frequency of turning patients.

e. Baccalaureate and associate degree nurses differ in use of touch as a thera-peutic device with patients.

5. Below are five simple hypotheses. Change each one to a complex hypothesis by adding either a dependent variable or an independent variable.

Simple Hypothesis   *Complex Hypothesis*

a. First-time blood donors experience greater stress during the donation than donors who have given blood previously.

b. Nurses who initiate more conversation with patients are rated more effective in their nursing care by patients than those who initiate less conversation.

c. Surgical patients who give high ratings to the informativeness of nursing communi-cations experience less preoperative stress than do patients who give low rat-ings.

d. Appendectomy patients whose perito-neums are drained with a Penrose drain experience more peritoneal infection than patients who are not drained.

e. Women who give birth by cesarean sec-tion are more likely to experience post-partum depression than women who give birth vaginally.

6. In Study Questions 4 and 5, 10 research hypotheses were provided. Identify the independent and dependent variables in each.

Independent Variable(s)   *Dependent Variable(s)*

4a. _____   _____
4b. _____   _____
4c. _____   _____
4d. _____   _____
4e. _____   _____
5a. _____   _____
5b. _____   _____
5c. _____   _____
5d. _____   _____
5e. _____   _____

7. Below are five statements that are not research hypotheses as currently stated. Suggest modifications to these statements that would make them testable research hypotheses.

Original Statement   *Hypothesis*

a. Relaxation therapy is effective in reducing hypertension.
b. The use of bilingual health care staff produces high utilization rates of health care facilities by ethnic minorities.
c. Nursing students are affected in their choice of clinical specialization by interactions with nursing faculty.
d. Sexually active teenagers have a high rate of using male methods of contraception.
e. In-use intravenous solutions become contaminated within 48 hours.

▍ D. APPLICATION EXERCISES

1. Woods (1993)* was interested in studying the notes made by various members of the health care team on patients' hospital charts. The investigator was concerned with several aspects of the chart in terms of its communication potential to various hospital personnel. She began her project with some general questions, such as: Are the nurses' entries on the patient chart used by other

_____
*This example is fictitious.

staff? Who is most likely to read nurses' entries on the patient chart? Are there particular types of medical conditions that encourage staff utilization of nurses' entries? Do particular types of entries encourage utilization?

Woods proceeded to reflect on her own experiences and observations relative to these issues and reviewed the literature to find whether other researchers had these problems. Based on her review and reflections, Woods developed the following hypotheses:

- Nursing notes on patients' charts are referred to infrequently by hospital personnel.
- Physicians refer to nursing notes on the patients' charts less frequently than do other personnel.
- The use of nursing notes by physicians is related to the location of the notes on the chart.
- Nurses perceive that nursing notes are referred to less frequently than they are in fact referred to.
- Nursing notes are more likely to be referred to by hospital personnel if the patient has been hospitalized for more than 5 days than if the patient has been hospitalized for 5 days or fewer.

Review and critique these hypotheses. Suggest alternative wordings or supplementary hypotheses. To assist you, here are some guiding questions (see also the questions in Box 4-2 of the text):

a. Are all the hypotheses testable as stated? What changes (if any) are needed to make all the hypotheses testable?

b. Are the hypotheses all consistent in format and style? That is, are they directional, nondirectional, or stated in the null form? Suggest changes, if appropriate, that would make them consistent.

c. Are the hypotheses reasonable (*i.e.,* logical and consistent with your own experience and observations)? Are the hypotheses significant (*i.e.,* do they have the potential to contribute to the nursing profession)?

d. Based on the general problem that the researcher identified, can you generate additional hypotheses that could be tested? Can you suggest modifications to the hypotheses to make them complex rather than simple (*i.e.,* introduce additional independent or dependent variables)?

2. Below are several suggested research articles. Read the introductory sections of one or more of these articles and identify the problem statement and hypotheses. Respond to parts **a** to **d** of Question D.1 in terms of these actual research studies and also answer relevant questions from Box 4-1 and Box 4-2 of the textbook.

- Deiriggi, P. M. (1990). Effects of waterbed flotation on indicators of energy expenditure in preterm infants. *Nursing Research, 39,* 140–146.
- Howell, R. D., MacRae, L. D., Sanjines, S., Burke, J., & DeStefano, P. (1992). Effects of two types of head coverings in the rewarming of patients after coronary artery bypass graft surgery. *Heart and Lung, 21,* 1–5.

- Maikler, V. E. (1991). Effects of a skin refrigerant/anesthetic and age on the pain responses of infants receiving immunizations. *Research in Nursing and Health, 14,* 397–402.
- Nyamathi, A., Jacoby, A., Constancia, P., & Ruvevich, S. (1992). Coping and adjustment of spouses of critically ill patients with cardiac disease. *Heart and Lung, 21,* 160–166.
- Van Riper, M., Ryff, C., & Pridham, K. (1992). Parental and family well-being in families of children with Down syndrome: A comparative study. *Research in Nursing and Health, 15,* 227–235.

3. Examine a recent issue of a nursing research journal. Find a research report that does not specify the research problem within the first two paragraphs. Rewrite the first two paragraphs to include a statement of the research problem.

4. Examine a recent issue of a nursing research journal. Find an article that fails to state a hypothesis. Given the research questions or problem statements that are included in the article, can you generate one or more hypotheses?

▌ E. SPECIAL PROJECTS

1. Read the article by Kuhlman and her colleagues (1991) entitled "Alzheimer's disease and family caregiving: Critical synthesis of the literature and research agenda," in *Nursing Research,* volume 40, issue 6 (or read some other research review article). Based on the author's summary of prior research, develop a problem statement for a study that would extend our knowledge about Alzheimer's disease family caregiving. Assess your problem statement in terms of the criteria discussed in Chapter 4 of the textbook.

2. Below are five general topics that could be investigated. Develop at least one problem statement for each. Assess the problem statement in terms of the criteria discussed in Chapter 4. If possible, develop a hypothesis based on the problem statement.

    a. Nurse–patient interaction: _____

    _____

    _____

    b. Bereavement: _____

    _____

    _____

    c. Nurses' diagnostic accuracy: _____

    _____

    _____

    d. Preoperative anxiety: _____

    _____

    _____

e. Sleep disturbances: _____

_____

_____

3. Below are two sets of variables. Select a variable from each set to generate directional hypotheses. In other words, use one variable in Set A as the independent variable and one variable in Set B as the dependent variable (or vice versa), and make a prediction about the relationship between the two.* Generate five hypotheses in this fashion.

Set A	*Set B*
Body temperature	Patient satisfaction with nursing care
Level of hopefulness	Regular versus no exercise
Attitudes toward death	Infant Apgar score
Frequency of medications	Patient gender
Delivery by nurse midwife versus physician	Effectiveness of nursing care
Participation in prenatal education classes	Patient capacity for self-care
Blood pressure	Patients' compliance with nursing instructions
Amount of interaction between nurses and patients' families	Amount of pain
Preoperative anxiety levels	Breast feeding duration
Patients' amount of privacy during hospitalization	Nurses' empathy
Smoking versus nonsmoking	Patients' pulse rates
Recidivism in a psychiatric hospital	Length of stay in hospital

---

*As one example: Pregnant women who smoke will give birth to babies with lower Apgar scores than women who do not smoke.

IIIIII Chapter 5
Theoretical Frameworks for Nursing Research

II A. MATCHING EXERCISES

1. Match each statement from Set B with one of the phrases in Set A. Indicate the letter corresponding to your response next to each of the statements in Set B.

Set A

a. Theory
b. Conceptual framework
c. Schematic model
d. Neither a, b, nor c
e. a, b, and c

Set B   *Responses*

1. Makes minimal use of language   _____
2. Uses concepts as building blocks   _____
3. Is essential in the conduct of good research   _____
4. Can be used as a basis for generating hypotheses   _____
5. Can be proved through empirical testing   _____
6. Indicates a system of propositions that assert relationships among variables   _____
7. Consists of interrelated concepts organized in a rational scheme but does not specify formal relationships among the concepts   _____
8. Exists in nature and is awaiting scientific discovery _____

2. Match each model from Set B with one of the nurse theorists in Set A. Indicate the letter corresponding to your response next to each of the statements in Set B.

Set A

a. Orem
b. Pender
c. Levine

d. Parse
e. Rogers
f. Roy

Set B   *Response*

1. Model of the Unitary Person   _____
2. Conservation Model   _____
3. Model of Man–Living–Health   _____
4. Model of Self-Care   _____
5. Adaptation Model   _____
6. Health Promotion Model   _____

▌ B. COMPLETION EXERCISES

Write the words or phrases that correctly complete the sentences below.

1. Theories are not found by scientists, they are _____ .
2. Deductions from theories are referred to as _____ .
3. Most of the conceptualizations of nursing practice would be called _____

   _____ .
4. Schematic models attempt to represent reality with a minimal use of _____

   _____ .
5. The four central concepts of conceptual models in nursing are _____ ,

   _____ , _____

   _____ , and _____ .
6. The acronym HBM stands for the _____ .
7. Theoretical frameworks from nonnursing disciplines are sometimes referred to

   as _____ .

▌ C. STUDY QUESTIONS

1. Define the following terms. Use the textbook to compare your definition with
   the definition in Chapter 5 or in the Glossary.

   a. Theory: _____

   _____

   _____

   b. Conceptual framework: _____

   _____

   _____

   c. Schematic model: _____

   _____

   _____

2. Read some recent issues of *Nursing Research* or another nursing research journal. Identify at least two different theories cited by nurse researchers in these research reports.

3. Choose one of the eight conceptual frameworks of nursing that were described in this chapter. Develop a research hypothesis based on this framework.

4. Select one of the problem statements listed in Question C.3 from Chapter 4 of this Study Guide. Could your selected problem be developed within one of the eight nursing frameworks discussed in this chapter? Defend your answer.

▌ D. APPLICATION EXERCISES

1. Sterling (1993)* developed a study derived from Rotter's social learning theory. Social learning theory postulates that human behaviors are contingent on the individual's expectancy that a particular behavior will be reinforced (rewarded). A key concept is locus of control, which is conceptualized as the degree to which a person perceives that rewards are a function of his or her own actions as opposed to external forces. Internal controllers are those who perceive themselves and their behaviors as the major determinants of the reinforcement, while external controllers are those who tend to see little, if any, relationship between their own actions and subsequent reinforcement.

_____

*This example is fictitious.

Sterling hypothesized that people with an internal locus-of-control orientation would be more likely to engage in preventive health care activities than those with an external orientation. As a rationale for this hypothesis, she reasoned that internally oriented people see themselves as capable of controlling health outcomes, whereas externally oriented people see forces outside their control as the major determinants of health outcomes. Therefore, the externally oriented are less likely to engage in preventive health care behaviors. To test her hypothesis, Sterling operationalized "willingness to engage in preventive health care activities" as enrollment in a health maintenance organization among a group of employees who were offered a choice between a traditional medical benefits package and HMO membership. Five hundred employees hired by a large industrial firm were administered a test that measured locus of control as part of the application process. Each new employee was offered a choice between the two medical programs. The 187 employees who chose HMO membership were found to have significantly higher (*i.e.,* more internal) scores on the locus-of-control measure than the 313 employees who elected the traditional medical plan, thereby supporting Sterling's hypothesis.

Review and critique the above study, particularly with respect to its theoretical basis. To assist you in this task, you can answer the guiding questions below as well as the questions in Box 5-1 of the text.

a. In what way, if any, did the use of a theory enhance the value of this study? Compare the meaningfulness of the study as described with what it would have been had the same hypothesis been tested in the absence of a theory.

b. In what way, if any, did the outcome of the study affect the value of the theory? If the outcome had been different (*e.g.,* no differences, or differences opposite to those predicted), what effect would that have had on the theory?

c. In the textbook, alternative ways of linking theory and research were described. In this example, how was the theory linked to the research?

2. Read the introductory sections of one of the actual research studies cited below. Apply parts **a** to **c** of Question D.1 to one of these studies as well as the questions in Box 5-1 of the textbook.

- Brown, S. J. (1992). Tailoring nursing care to the individual client: Empirical challenge of a theoretical concept. *Research in Nursing and Health, 15,* 39–46.

- Cupples, S. A. (1991). Effects of timing and reinforcement of preoperative education on knowledge and recovery of patients having coronary artery bypass graft surgery. *Heart and Lung, 20,* 654–660.

- Huss, K. Sr., Salerno, M., & Huss, R. W. (1991). Computer-assisted reinforcement of instruction: Effects on adherence in adult atopic asthmatics. *Research in Nursing and Health, 14,* 259–267.

- McClowry, S. G. (1990). The relationship of temperament to pre- and post-hospitalized behavioral responses of school-age children. *Nursing Research, 39*, 30–35.
- Redeker, N. S. (1992). The relationship between uncertainty and coping after coronary bypass surgery. *Western Journal of Nursing Research, 14*, 48–68.

‖ E. SPECIAL PROJECTS

1. One proposition of reinforcement theory is that *if* a behavior is rewarded (reinforced), *then* the behavior will be repeated (learned). Based on this theory and on your observation of behaviors in health settings or schools of nursing, suggest three nursing research problem statements.
2. Develop a researchable problem statement based on Orem's Model of Self-Care.

Designs for Nursing Research

Part III

▌▌▌▌▌▌ Chapter 6
Research Design

▌ A. MATCHING EXERCISES

1. Match each problem statement from Set B with one (or more) of the phrases from Set A that indicates a potential reason for using a nonexperimental approach. Indicate the letter(s) corresponding to your response next to each statement in Set B.

Set A

a. Independent variable cannot be manipulated
b. Ethical constraints on manipulation
c. Practical constraints on manipulation
d. No constraints on manipulation

Set B   *Responses*

1. Does the use of certain tampons cause toxic shock syndrome? _____
2. Does heroin addiction among mothers affect the Apgar scores of their infants? _____
3. Is the age of a hemodialysis patient related to the incidence of the disequilibrium syndrome? _____
4. What body positions aid respiratory function? _____
5. Does the ingestion of saccharin cause cancer in humans? _____
6. Is a nurse's attitude toward the elderly related to his or her choice of a clinical specialty? _____
7. Does the use of touch by nursing staff affect patient morale? _____
8. Does a nurse's gender affect his or her salary and rate of promotion? _____
9. Does extreme athletic exertion in young women cause amenorrhea? _____
10. Does assertiveness training affect a psychiatric nurse's job performance? _____

2. Match each problem statement from Set B with one (or more) of the types of research listed in Set A. Indicate the letter(s) corresponding to your response next to each of the statements in Set B.

Set A

a. Survey research
b. Evaluation research
c. Field study
d. Historical research

e. Case study
f. Methodologic research
g. Needs assessment

Set B   *Responses*

1. What types of social and health service are needed by the rural elderly? _____

2. Does the assurance of anonymity to respondents increase self-reports of socially undesirable behavior, such as child or spouse abuse? _____

3. Do parents approve of sex education in the schools? _____

4. Does an intervention designed to provoke laughter reduce anxiety in hospitalized children? _____

5. Has the image of male nurses changed over time? _____

6. How do the elderly in a nursing home react toward the death of another nursing home resident? _____

7. Is a radio-based media campaign more effective than a print-based media campaign in recruiting blood donors? _____

8. How does a community react to the stress of a natural disaster, such as a hurricane? _____

9. How does the general public feel about euthanasia? _____

10. Does the block-rotation method of scheduling result in a lower absentee rate among nursing staff than a random rotation method? _____

▐ B. COMPLETION EXERCISES

Write the words or phrases that correctly complete the sentences below.

1. In an experiment, the researcher manipulates the _____ variable.

2. The manipulation that the researcher introduces is referred to as the experimental _____ .

3. Randomization is performed so that groups will be formed without _____ _____ .

4. When more than one independent variable is being simultaneously manipulated by the researcher, the design is referred to as a(n) _____ .

5. Each factor in an experimental design must have two or more _____ .

6. Subjects serve as their own controls in a(n) _____ design.

7. A primary objective of a true experiment is to enable the researcher to infer _____ .

8. When a true experimental design is not used, the control group is usually referred to as the _____ group.

9. A research design that involves a manipulation but lacks the controls of a quasi-experiment is referred to as a(n) _____ design.

10. A quasi-experimental design that involves repeated observations over time is referred to as a(n) _____ design.

11. When data are gathered before the institution of treatment, the initial data gathering is referred to as the _____ .

12. When neither the subjects nor the people collecting data know in which group a subject is participating, the procedures are called _____ .

13. When no variable is manipulated in a study, the research is called _____ .

14. In ex post facto research, the investigator forfeits control over the _____ variable.

15. In ex post facto research, it is difficult, if not impossible, to establish _____ relationships.

16. A prospective design is more rigorous in elucidating causal relations than a _____ design.

17. When data are collected at more than one point in time, the design is referred to as _____ .

18. Longitudinal studies conducted to determine the long-term outcomes of some condition or intervention are called _____ .

19. The type of study that collects extensive self-report information on people's attitudes, actions, beliefs, and intentions is called _____ .

20. Intensive studies in naturalistic social settings are referred to as _____ .

21. The effectiveness of a policy or program is studied in a(n) _____ .

22. The method of collecting needs assessment data by questioning knowledgeable people is known as the _____ approach.

23. Methodologic research is research conducted for the purpose of developing or refining research _____ .

24. The environment should be controlled by the researcher insofar as possible by maximizing _____ in research conditions.

25. The specifications of an experimental treatment are often referred to as the research _____ .

26. Using the principle of homogeneity to control extraneous variables limits the _____ of the findings.

27. The research procedure that controls all possible extraneous variables when two or more groups are involved is known as _____ .

28. Control over extraneous variables is required for the _____ validity of the study.

29. The differential loss of subjects from comparison groups is the threat known as

_____ .

30. Changes that occur as the result of time passing rather than as a result of the effects of the independent variable represent the threat of _____

_____ .

‖ C. STUDY QUESTIONS

1. Define the following terms. Use the textbook to compare your definition with the definition in Chapter 6 or in the Glossary.

   a. Experimental: _____

   _____

   _____

   b. Manipulation: _____

   _____

   _____

   c. Randomization: _____

   _____

   _____

   d. Control group: _____

   _____

   _____

  e. Double-blind experiment: _____

_____

_____

  f. Interaction effects: _____

_____

_____

  g. Hawthorne effect: _____

_____

_____

  h. Quasi-experimental design: _____

_____

_____

  i. Ex post facto research: _____

_____

_____

  j. Retrospective study: _____

_____

_____

  k. Prospective study: _____

_____

_____

  l. Nonexperimental research: _____

_____

_____

  m. Cross-sectional study: _____

_____

_____

  n. Trend study: _____

_____

_____

  o. Panel study: _____

_____

_____

  p. Case study: _____

_____

_____

q. Historical research: _____

_____

_____

r. Randomized block design: _____

_____

_____

s. Matching: _____

_____

_____

t. Internal validity: _____

_____

_____

u. Selection threat: _____

_____

_____

v. Attrition: _____

_____

_____

w. External validity: _____

_____

_____

x. Clinical trial: _____

_____

_____

y. Case control study: _____

_____

_____

z. Crossover design: _____

_____

_____

2. Which of the following variables are *inherently* not amenable to research manipulation?*

	Can Be Manipulated	Cannot Be Manipulated
a. Age at onset of obesity		
b. Amount of auditory stimulation		
c. Number of cigarettes smoked		
d. Infant's birth weight		
e. Blood type		
f. Preoperative anxiety		
g. Amount and timing of endotracheal suctioning		
h. Attitudes toward abortion		
i. Nurses' shift assignment		
j. Method of birth control used		
k. Mother–infant bonding		
l. Use of A-V shunt versus A-V fistula		
m. Amount of fluid intake		
n. Morale of AIDS patients		
o. Frequency of turning patients		

3. A nurse researcher found a relationship between teenagers' level of knowledge about birth control and their level of sexual activity. That is, teenagers with higher levels of sexual activity know more about birth control than teenagers with less sexual activity. Suggest at least three interpretations for this finding:

a. _____

_____

_____

b. _____

_____

_____

c. _____

_____

_____

Manipulation does not mean that the variable can be *affected* by a researcher; it refers to the researcher's ability to randomly assign people to different levels of the variable or to different groups.

Does this research situation describe a research problem that is *inherently* nonexperimental? Why or why not?

4. A researcher has found that supervisors' ratings of nurses' job performance are related to the nurses' self-reported job satisfaction. That is, nurses who received better job evaluations were more satisfied with their jobs than nurses with lower ratings. Suggest at least three interpretations for this result.

a. _____

_____

_____

b. _____

_____

_____

c. _____

_____

_____

Does this research situation describe a research problem that is *inherently* nonexperimental? Why or why not?

5. Refer to the 10 hypotheses in Questions C.4 and C.5 of Chapter 4. Indicate below whether these hypotheses could be tested using an experimental or quasi-experimental approach, a nonexperimental approach, or both.

Experimental or Quasi-Experimental	*Nonexperimental*	*Both*
4a. ——	——	——
4b. ——	——	——
4c. ——	——	——
4d. ——	——	——
4e. ——	——	——
5a. ——	——	——
5b. ——	——	——
5c. ——	——	——
5d. ——	——	——
5e. ——	——	——

6. Examine the 10 problem statements in the first matching exercise of this chapter. For each, specify one or more extraneous variables that the researcher might want to control.

1. _____

2. _____

3. _____

4. _____

5. _____

6. _____

7. _____

8. _____

9. _____

10. _____

7. A nurse researcher is interested in comparing the oral and rectal temperature measurements of febrile adults two times a day on three different wards. Could such a study be conducted as a factorial experiment? Why or why not? If yes, what are the factors in the design? Could a randomized block design be used? Why or why not? If yes, what would the blocking variable(s) be?

8. Suppose you wanted to evaluate the effect of an experimental approach to teaching student nurses how to give subcutaneous injections. In conducting a true experiment for this study, what environmental factors would you want to control to maintain the constancy of research conditions?

9. Place a check next to those types of research below that are *inherently* nonexperimental:

    a. Survey research   _____

    b. Evaluation research   _____

    c. Needs assessments   _____

    d. Case studies   _____

    e. Field research   _____

    f. Historical research   _____

    g. Methodologic research   _____

10. Below are several research problems. Indicate for each whether you think the problem should be studied using a survey approach or a field study approach. Justify your response.

a. By what process do new nursing home residents learn to adapt to their environments?

_____

_____

b. To what extent are dietary habits and exercise patterns in healthy adults related?

_____

_____

c. What is the relationship between a teenager's health-risk appraisal and various forms of risk-taking behavior (*e.g.*, smoking, sexual activity without contraception, using drugs, etc.)?

_____

_____

d. What aspects of the lifestyles of urban disadvantaged women place them at especially high risk of pregnancy and childbirth complications?

_____

_____

e. How are the dynamics of nurse–patient interaction affected by the presence of a physician?

_____

_____

‖ D. APPLICATION EXERCISES

1. Koshgarian (1993)† wanted to test the effectiveness of a new relaxation and biofeedback intervention on menopause symptoms. She invited women who presented themselves in an outpatient clinic with complaints of severe hot flashes to participate in the study of the experimental treatment. These 30 women were asked to record, every day for 1 week before their treatment, the frequency and duration of their hot flashes. During the intervention, which

_____

†This example is fictitious.

involved six 1-hour sessions over a 3-week period, the women again recorded their symptoms. Then, 4 weeks after the treatment, the women were asked to record their hot flashes over a 5-day period. At the end of the study, Koshgarian found that both the frequency and average duration of the hot flashes had been significantly reduced in this sample of women. She concluded that her new treatment was an effective alternative to estrogen replacement therapy in treating menopausal hot flashes.

Review and critique this study. Suggest alternative designs for testing the effectiveness of the treatment. To assist you in your critique, here are some guiding questions. (See also the critiquing guidelines in Box 6-1 of the textbook.)

a. Is the design of this study experimental, quasi-experimental, preexperimental, or nonexperimental?

b. Evaluate the internal validity of the study. Does the design eliminate or minimize the threat of history? selection? maturation? mortality?

c. The investigator concluded that the outcome (*i.e.,* the reduction in the frequency and duration of the women's hot flashes) was attributable to the treatment. Can you offer one or more alternative explanations to account for the outcome?

d. Consider your responses to parts **b** and **c** above. If you have identified any weaknesses in the design of this research, suggest a modified design that would improve the internal validity of the study. In what way does your new design eliminate the problems of the original design? Have you dealt with all the threats to the study's internal validity?

e. Does this study fall into a category described in the section of the chapter on additional types of research (*i.e.,* is it a survey, field study, etc.)?

2. Below are several suggested research articles. Read the introductory and methods sections of one or more of these articles and respond to parts **a** to **e** from Question D.1 in terms of these actual research studies.

- Ganong, L. H. & Coleman, M. (1992). The effect of clients' family structure on nursing students' cognitive schemas and verbal behavior. *Research in Nursing & Health, 15,* 139–146.

- Gulick, E. E. (1991). Self-assessed health and use of health services. *Western Journal of Nursing Research, 13,* 195–211.

- Liehr, P., Todd, B., Rossi, M., & Culligan, M. (1992). Effect of venous support on edema and leg pain in patients after coronary artery bypass graft surgery. *Heart and Lung, 21,* 6–11.

- McCain, G. C. (1992). Facilitating inactive awake states in preterm infants: A study of three interventions. *Nursing Research, 41,* 157–160.

- Weinbacher, F. M., Littlejohn, C. E., & Conley, P. F. (1990). Growth of bacteria in prefilled syringes stored in home refrigerators. *Applied Nursing Research, 3,* 63–67.

3. Roche (1992)‡ hypothesized that the absence of socioemotional supports among the elderly results in a high level of chronic health problems and low morale. She tested this hypothesis by interviewing a sample of 250 residents of one community who were aged 65 and older. The respondents were randomly selected from a list of town residents. Roche used several measures of the availability of socioemotional supports: (1) whether the respondent lived with any kin; (2) whether the respondent had any living children who resided within 30 minutes away; (3) the total number of interactions the respondent had had in the previous week with kin not residing in his or her household; and (4) the number of close friends in whom the respondent felt he or she could confide. Based on responses to the various questions on social support, respondents were classified in one of three groups: low social support, moderate social support, and high social support. In a 6-month follow-up interview, Roche collected information from 214 respondents about the frequency and intensity of the respondents' illnesses in the preceding 6 months, their hospitalization records, their overall satisfaction with life, and their attitudes toward their own aging. An analysis of the data revealed that the low-support group had significantly more health problems, lower life satisfaction ratings, and lower acceptance of their aging than the other two groups. Roche concluded that the availability of social supports resulted in better physical and mental adjustment to old age.

Review and critique this study. Suggest alternative designs for testing the researcher's hypotheses. To assist you in your critique, here are some guiding questions. (See also the critiquing guidelines in Box 6-1 of the textbook.)

   a. Is the design described above experimental, quasi-experimental, preexperimental, or nonexperimental? If it is nonexperimental, is it inherently so? Why or why not?
   b. Evaluate the internal validity of the study. What threats to its internal validity, if any, are posed?
   c. Examine the criteria for causality presented in Chapter 6 of the textbook. Does this study meet all the criteria for establishing causality?
   d. The researcher concluded that her independent variable (amount of social support) "caused" certain outcomes (mental and physical health status in the elderly). Can you offer two or more alternative explanations to account for the findings?
   e. Consider your responses to parts **b** through **d** above. If you have identified any weaknesses in the design of the research, suggest modifications that would improve the internal validity of the study.
   f. Does this study fall into a category described in the section of the chapter on additional types of research (*i.e.*, is it a survey, field study, etc.)?

---

‡This example is fictitious.

4. Below are several suggested research articles. Read the introductory and methods sections of one or more of these articles and respond to parts **a** to **f** of Question D.3 above in terms of these actual research studies.

- Covington, C., Cronenwett, L., & Loveland-Cherry, C. (1991). Newborn behavioral performance in colic and non-colic infants. *Nursing Research, 40,* 292–296.
- Hill, P. D., & Aldag, J. (1991). Potential indicators of insufficient milk supply syndrome. *Research in Nursing and Health, 14,* 11–19.
- Keltner, B., Keltner, N. L., & Farren, E. (1990). Family routines and conduct disorders in adolescent girls. *Western Journal of Nursing Research, 12,* 161–174.
- Monsen, R. B. (1992). Autonomy, coping, and self-care agency in healthy adolescents and in adolescents with spina bifida. *Journal of Pediatric Nursing, 7,* 9–13.
- Schraeder, B. D., Heverly, M. A., & Rappaport, J. (1990). Temperament, behavior problems, and learning skills in very low birth weight preschoolers. *Research in Nursing and Health, 13,* 27–34.

5. Roth (1993)§ investigated the relationship between the use of intrauterine devices (IUDs) and the incidence of pelvic inflammatory disease (PID) in a sample of urban women. The data were gathered from the gynecology departments of four health centers (one university, one city hospital, one health maintenance organization, and one consortium of private gynecologists). Roth obtained the records of 600 women—150 from each facility—who were diagnosed within the previous 12 months as having PID. She also obtained the records of 150 women who had come to each of the facilities for some other purpose and who had no record of having had PID within the 12-month period before their focal visit. The two groups of 600 women (the PID and non-PID group) were matched in terms of age (within 5-year ranges of 20 or under, 21 to 25, 26 to 30, 31 to 35 years old, etc.) and marital status (currently married or not married). For each of the 1200 women, the records were examined to determine whether they had had an IUD inserted within 2 years before their focal visit. For those women for whom no determination could be made based on the records of the facility, brief telephone interviews were administered to obtain the needed information (30 women who could not be reached were replaced with other women to maintain the sample size). The data revealed that 122 women in the PID group (20.3%), compared with 74 women in the non-PID group (12.3%), had used an IUD, a significant group difference. Based on this analysis, Roth concluded that use of an IUD was a causative factor of PID in this sample.

---

§This example is fictitious.

Review and critique this study. Suggest alternative designs for testing the researcher's hypotheses. To assist you in your critique, here are some guiding questions. (See also the critiquing guidelines in Box 6-1 of the textbook.)

   a. Apply parts **a** through **e** of Question D.3 to this current example.
   b. What extraneous variables did the researcher identify, and by what method were they controlled? How else might they have been controlled?
   c. What extraneous variables do you think *should* have been controlled but were not? Why might the researcher have decided not to control these variables?
   d. To what extent did the researcher control for the constancy of conditions in this study? Suggest ways in which this aspect of the study could have been improved.
   e. Evaluate the external validity of the study in terms of the threats described in Chapter 6 of the textbook. What changes, if any, would you recommend to improve the external validity of the design?
   f. Does this study fall into a category described in the section of the chapter on additional types of research (*i.e.*, is it a survey, field study, etc.)?

6. Below are several suggested research articles. Read the introductory and methods sections of one or more of these articles and respond to parts **a** to **f** of Question D.5 in terms of these actual research studies.

   ■ Beckmann, C. A. (1990). Postterm pregnancy: Effects on temperature and glucose regulation. *Nursing Research, 39,* 21–24.
   ■ DiIorio, C., Faherty, B., & Manteuffel, B. (1991). Cognitive-perceptual factors associated with antiepileptic medication compliance. *Research in Nursing and Health, 14,* 329–337.
   ■ Giuffre, M., Heidenreich, T., Carney-Gersten, P., Dorsch, J. A., & Heidenreich, E. (1990). The relationship between axillary and core body temperature measurements. *Applied Nursing Research, 3,* 52–55.
   ■ Wallston, K. A., Smith, R. A. P., King, J. E., Smith, M. S., Rye, P., & Burish, T. G. (1991). Desire for control and choice of antiemetic treatment for cancer chemotherapy. *Western Journal of Nursing Research, 13,* 12–21.

7. Schoen (1993) ‖ hypothesized that aging negatively affects intellectual capacity and motor responsivity. To test this hypothesis, she randomly selected the names of 250 men aged 70 or above; 250 men in their 50s; and 250 men in their 30s from the residents living in a mid-sized city in Illinois. Schoen realized that intellectual capacity is sometimes correlated with social class. Furthermore, mortality rates vary by social class. Therefore, the subjects were selected in such a way that half in each group were from lower-income households (household income $20,000 or less) and half were from higher-income

---

‖ This example is fictitious.

households (income over $20,000). The basic design for the analysis, therefore, was as follows:

	Age Group		
Income Group	**30s**	**50s**	**70s**
≤ $20,000			
> $20,000			

The 750 people were administered an intelligence test that measured verbal aptitude, problem solving, quantitative skills, spatial aptitude, and overall intelligence. In addition, the subjects were given various reaction-time tests. The analysis of the data revealed that, as hypothesized, intelligence declined with age in both income groups. Except on the measure of verbal aptitude, the subjects in their 30s scored highest, and the subjects in their 70s scored lowest on the subtest of intellectual capacity and on overall intelligence. The same pattern was observed for reaction time. Schoen concluded that the aging process causes deterioration of both intellectual and motor capacity.

Review and critique Schoen's study. Suggest alternative designs or other modifications for testing the researcher's hypothesis. Use parts **a** through **e** from Question D.5 to guide you in your critique. In addition, answer the following questions:
  a. Is this design cross-sectional or longitudinal?
  b. What problems, if any, does this design pose in terms of testing the hypothesis?
  c. What design, if any, might be more appropriate?
  d. What difficulties, if any, would Schoen have had in implementing your recommended design?
  e. Does this study fall into a category described in the section of the chapter on additional types of research (*i.e.,* is it a survey, field study, etc.)?
8. Below are several suggested research articles. Read the introductory and methods sections of one or more of these articles and respond to parts **a** through **e** of Question D.7 in terms of these actual research studies.
  ▪ Beach, E. K., Maloney, B. H., Plocica, A. R., Sherry, S. E., Weaver, M., Luthringer, L., & Utz, S. (1992). The spouse: A factor in recovery after acute myocardial infarction. *Heart and Lung, 21,* 30–38.
  ▪ Gennaro, S., & Stringer, M. (1991). Stress and health in low birthweight infants: A longitudinal study. *Nursing Research, 40,* 308–311.

- Hall, L. A., Gurley, D. N., Sachs, B., & Kryscio, R. J. (1991). Psychosocial predictors of maternal depressive symptoms, parenting attitudes, and child behavior in single-parent families. *Nursing Research, 40,* 214–220.
- Pridham, K. F., & Chang, A. S. (1991). Mothers' perceptions of problem-solving competence for infant care. *Western Journal of Nursing Research, 13,* 164–174.

▌ E. SPECIAL PROJECTS

1. Suppose that you were interested in testing the hypothesis that a regular regimen of exercise reduces blood pressure, improves cardiovascular efficiency, and increases coronary circulation. Design a quasi-experiment to test the hypothesis. Evaluate the design in regard to its internal validity. Design a true experiment to test the same hypothesis and compare the internal validity of this design with that of the quasi-experiment.

2. Suppose that you were interested in testing the hypothesis that the use of an IUD could cause infertility. Describe how such a hypothesis could be tested using a retrospective design. Now describe a prospective design for the same study. Compare the strengths and weaknesses of the two approaches. Could an experimental or quasi-experimental design be used? Why or why not?

3. Suppose that you wanted to compare premature and normal infants in terms of their development at age 5. Describe how you would design such a study, being careful to indicate what extraneous variables you would need to control and how you would control them.

4. Suppose that you were interested in testing the effect of packing sugar on a wound on the wound-healing process. Describe a design you would recommend for this problem, being careful to indicate what extraneous variables you would need to control and how you would control them.

5. Suppose that you were interested in studying short-term versus long-term impacts of the death of a spouse on the physical and mental health of the surviving spouse. Design a cross-sectional study to research the question, specifying the characteristics of your sample. Now design a longitudinal study for the same problem. Identify the advantages and disadvantages of the two designs.

6. Generate one problem statement for each of the seven types of research that were described in this chapter.

   a. Survey research: _____

   _____

   _____

   b. Field research: _____

   _____

   _____

c. Evaluation research: _____
    _____
    _____

d. Needs assessment: _____
    _____
    _____

e. Case study: _____
    _____
    _____

f. Historical research: _____
    _____
    _____

g. Methodologic research: _____
    _____
    _____

▌▊▊ Chapter 7
Sampling Designs

▌ A. MATCHING EXERCISES

1. Match each statement from Set B with one of the phrases from Set A. Indicate the letter corresponding to your response next to each of the statements in Set B.

Set A

a. Probability sampling
b. Nonprobability sampling
c. Both probability and nonprobability sampling
d. Neither probability nor nonprobability sampling

Set B   *Responses*

   1. Includes systematic sampling procedures   _____
   2. Allows an estimation of the magnitude of sampling error   _____
   3. Guarantees a representative sample   _____
   4. Includes quota sampling   _____
   5. Yields more accurate results when the samples are large   _____
   6. Elements are selected by nonrandom methods   _____
   7. Can be used with entire populations or with selected strata
       from the populations   _____
   8. Is used to select populations   _____
   9. Provides an equal chance of elements being selected   _____
  10. Is required when the population is homogeneous   _____

▌ B. COMPLETION EXERCISES

Write the words or phrases that correctly complete the sentences below.

1. A(n) _____ is a subset of the elements that comprise the population.

2. The main criterion for evaluating a sample is its _____ of the population being studied.

3. A sample would be considered _____ if it systematically overrepresented or underrepresented a segment of the population.

4. If a population is completely _____ with respect to key attributes, then any sample is as good as any other.

5. Another term used for convenience sample is _____ .

6. Quota samples are essentially convenience samples from selected _____ _____ of the population.

7. Another term for a purposive sample is a(n) _____ sample.

8. The most basic type of probability sampling is referred to as _____ _____ .

9. When disproportionate sampling is used, an adjustment procedure known as _____ is normally used to estimate population values.

10. Another term used to refer to cluster sampling is _____ sampling.

11. In systematic samples, the distance between selected elements is referred to as the _____ .

12. Differences between population values and sample values are referred to as _____ .

13. If a researcher has confidence in his or her sampling design, the results of a study can reasonably be generalized to the _____ population.

14. As the size of a sample _____ , the probability of drawing a deviant sample diminishes.

15. If a researcher wanted to draw a systematic sample of 100 from a population of 3000, the sampling interval would be _____ .

▮ C. STUDY QUESTIONS

1. Define the following terms. Use the textbook to compare your definition with the definition in Chapter 7 or in the Glossary.

a. Population: _____

_____

_____

b. Elements: _____

_____

_____

c. Probability sampling: _____

_____

_____

d. Nonprobability sampling: _____

_____

_____

e. Stratum: _____

_____

_____

f. Snowball sampling: _____

_____

_____

g. Quota sampling: _____

_____

_____

h. Purposive sampling: _____

_____

_____

i. Sampling frame: _____

_____

_____

j. Stratified random sampling: _____

_____

_____

k. Disproportionate sample: _____

_____

_____

l. Cluster sampling: _____

_____

_____

m. Systematic sampling: _____

_____

_____

n. Power analysis: _____

_____

_____

o. Response rate: _____

_____

_____

2. Identify the type of sampling design used in the following examples:

Type of Design

a. Thirty nursing faculty randomly sampled from a random selection of 10 nursing schools.   _____

b. All the nurses participating in a continuing education seminar.   _____

c. A sample of 250 members randomly selected from a roster of ANA members.   _____

d. Every 20th patient admitted to the emergency room in the month of June.   _____

e. The first 20 male and the first 20 female patients admitted to the hospital with hypothermia.   _____

f. Fifteen people known by the researcher to have hypertension and 15 people known not to have hypertension.   _____

g. Twenty-five people whose family members had attempted suicide, most of whom were referred by other members already in the sample.   _____

3. Suppose a researcher has decided to use a systematic sampling design for a research project. The known population size is 4400, and the sample size desired is 200. What is the sampling interval? If the first element selected is 112, what would be the second, third, and fourth elements to be selected?

4. Read the following article and identify what the successive clusters were in drawing the research sample: Yarcheski, A., & Mahan, N. E. (1985). The unification model in nursing. *Nursing Research, 34,* 120–125.

5. Suppose a researcher were interested in studying the smoking habits of nurses. Suggest a possible target and accessible population for a researcher working in your area. What strata might be identified by the researcher if quota sampling were used?

▌ D. APPLICATION EXERCISES

1. Dresser (1993)* studied the job-search strategies of recent nursing school graduates. Her survey focused on such issues as timing of job applications, number of applications, source of information about jobs, method of initial contact, and so on. She was interested in learning whether certain strategies were more successful in achieving job offers than others. She obtained lists of graduates from six schools of nursing in the Washington, DC area (two schools for each of three different types of programs). She then conducted telephone interviews with 100 graduates from each of the three program types (bachelors, diploma, and associates). Her method was to find, using local telephone directories and directory assistance, the telephone numbers for as many of the names on her lists as she could and to make calls until she had completed 100 interviews with graduates from each group. Thus, her final sample consisted of 300 recently graduated RNs.

Review and critique this research effort. Suggest alternative sampling designs. To assist you in your critique, use the questions below as well as the questions in Box 7-1 of the text.
   a. What type of sampling design was used? Was this design appropriate? Would you recommend a different sampling approach? Why or why not? What are the advantages of the approach used? The disadvantages?
   b. Identify what you believe to be the target and accessible populations in this study. How representative do you feel the accessible population is of the target population? How representative is the sample of this accessible population? What are some of the possible sources of sampling bias?
   c. Did the research use a proportionate or disproportionate sampling plan? Is this appropriate? Why or why not?
   d. Comment on the size of the sample. Does this sample size appear to be adequate?

---

*This example is fictitious.

2. Below are several suggested research articles. Read the introductory and methods sections of one or more of these articles and respond to parts **a** through **d** of Question D.1 in terms of these actual research studies.
   - Burman, M. E. (1992). The organizational environments and services of VNAs and hospital-based home health care agencies. *Research in Nursing and Health, 15,* 285–294.
   - Korniewicz, D. M., Kirwin, M., Cresci, K., Markut, C., & Larson, E. (1992). In-use comparison of latex gloves in two high-risk units. *Heart and Lung, 21,* 81–84.
   - Macnee, C. L. (1991). Perceived well-being of persons quitting smoking. *Nursing Research, 40,* 200–203.
   - Rustia, J., & Abbott, D. A. (1990). Predicting paternal role enactment. *Western Journal of Nursing Research, 12,* 145–160.
   - Sulzbach, L. M., & Munro, B. H. (1991). Survey of nursing practice related to decanting intravenous solutions. *Heart and Lung, 20,* 624–630.

▌ E. SPECIAL PROJECTS

1. Suppose that you were interested in studying preventive health care behaviors among low-income urban residents. Describe how you might select a sample for your study using the following:
   a. An accidental sample
   b. A quota sample
   c. A cluster sample
2. Propose a researchable problem statement. Specify a research and sampling design to study this problem. In particular, specify the following:
   a. The target population, including all criteria for inclusion in the population
   b. An accessible population
   c. A sampling design, together with a rationale
   d. A recommended sample size

   With respect to **b** through **d**, be realistic. Take into account available resources, time, and level of expertise. That is, recommend a plan that would be feasible to implement.

Collection of Research Data

Part IV

IIIIIII Chapter 8
Methods of Data Collection

II A. MATCHING EXERCISES

1. Match each descriptive statement from Set B with one of the statements from Set A. Indicate the letter corresponding to your response next to each item in Set B.

Set A

a. An interview schedule
b. A questionnaire
c. Both an interview schedule and a questionnaire
d. Neither an interview schedule nor a questionnaire

Set B   Responses

1. Can provide respondents with the protection of anonymity   _____
2. Can be used with illiterate respondents   _____
3. Can contain both open- and closed-ended questions   _____
4. Is used in survey research   _____
5. Is the best way to measure human behavior   _____
6. Generally has high response rates   _____
7. Is generally an inexpensive method of data collection   _____
8. Benefits from pretesting   _____

2. Match each descriptive statement from Set B with one (or more) of the statements from Set A. Indicate the letter(s) corresponding to your response next to each item in Set B.

Set A

a. Likert scales
b. Semantic differential scales
c. Neither a nor b

Set B   *Responses*

1. Provides a quantitative measure of an attribute   _____
2. Can be used to measure attitudes   _____
3. Is sometimes referred to as a summated rating scale   _____
4. Is subject to response set biases   _____
5. Is often used to measure behavioral characteristics   _____
6. Presents statements to which respondents indicate agreement
   or disagreement   _____
7. Rarely contains more than five items   _____
8. Uses a graphic rating scale format   _____

3. Match each problem statement from Set B with one of the statements from Set A. Indicate the letter corresponding to your response next to each item in Set B.

Set A

a. The study would *require* observational data.
b. The study *could* use observational data, as well as other forms of data.
c. The study is not amenable to observational data collection.

Set B   *Responses*

1. Are nurses' attitudes toward abortion related to their years of nursing experience?   _____
2. Are patients' levels of stress related to their willingness to disclose their own fears to nursing staff?   _____
3. Are the crying patterns of infants related to their gestational age at birth?   _____
4. Is the degree of physical activity of a psychiatric patient related to his or her length of hospitalization?   _____
5. Are first-year nurses' ratings of effectiveness more highly related to their clinical grades or to their grades in academic courses while in nursing school?   _____
6. Is a child's fear during immunization related to the nurse's method of preparing the child for the shot?   _____
7. Does the presence of the father in the delivery room affect the mother's level of pain?   _____
8. Is the ability of dialysis patients to cleanse and dress their shunts related to their self-esteem?   _____
9. Is compliance with a medication regimen higher among women than men?   _____
10. Is aggressive behavior among hospitalized mentally retarded children related to styles of discipline by hospital staff?   _____

▍▍ B. COMPLETION EXERCISES

Write the words or phrases that correctly complete the sentences below.

1. The four dimensions along which data collection methods can vary are _____

   _____ , _____ ,

   _____ , and _____ .

2. Subjects in self-report studies are often referred to as _____

   _____ or _____ .

3. In a focused interview, general question areas are normally prepared in the form

   of a _____ .

4. When several respondents are assembled in one place to discuss questions, the

   approach being used is referred to as a _____ .

5. A disadvantage of _____ questions is that

   the researcher may inadvertently omit some potentially important alternatives.

6. _____ questions are relatively inefficient in

   terms of the respondents' time.

7. If respondents are not very verbal or articulate, _____

   questions are generally most appropriate.

8. Nonresponse in self-report studies is generally not _____

   and can therefore lead to bias.

9. A _____ is a device designed to assign

   scores to subjects in order to discriminate among them with respect to an at-

   tribute of interest.

10. Likert scales consist of a number of statements written in the _____

    _____ form.

11. In Likert scales, positively worded statements are scored in one direction, and

    the scoring of negatively worded statements is _____ .

12. With a semantic differential, subjects are asked to rate concepts on a series of

    _____ .

13. The bias introduced when respondents select options at either end of the re-

    sponse continuum is known as _____ .

14. The major focus of observation in nursing research is on human _____

    _____ .

15. The problem of behavioral distortions arising when subjects are aware that they

    are being observed is known as _____ .

16. The technique known as _____ involves the

    collection of unstructured observational data while the researcher participates

    in the activities of the group being observed.

17. The three major types of observational positioning in participant observation studies are _____ , _____ , and _____ positioning.

18. Data from unstructured observations are generally recorded on _____ _____ and _____ .

19. In a structured observational setting, the most common procedure is to construct a(n) _____ for observed behaviors.

20. One of the major difficulties with observational data is the possibility that the observers are not _____ .

21. Biophysiologic measures that are taken directly within a living organism are _____ measures.

22. When physiologic materials are extracted from subjects and subjected to analysis, the data are referred to as _____ measures.

23. The major advantage of using existing records is that they are _____ _____ .

24. In Q sorts, forcing subjects to place a predetermined number of cards in each pile helps eliminate _____ _____ .

25. The Rorschach test is an example of a _____ technique.

26. Critics of projective techniques claim that these methods are incapable of objective _____ .

27. _____ are brief narrative descriptions of people or situations to which subjects are asked to react.

▌ C. STUDY QUESTIONS

1. Define the following terms. Use the textbook to compare your definition with the definition in Chapter 8 or in the Glossary.

a. Unstructured interview: _____
_____
_____

b. Focused interview: _____
_____
_____

c. Interview schedule: _____
_____
_____

d. Questionnaire: _____
_____
_____

e. Probe: _____

_____

_____

f. Scale: _____

_____

_____

g. Likert scale: _____

_____

_____

h. Semantic differential: _____

_____

_____

i. Visual analog scale: _____

_____

_____

j. Response set biases: _____

_____

_____

k. Social desirability response bias: _____

_____

_____

l. Acquiescence response set bias: _____

_____

_____

m. Reactivity: _____

_____

_____

n. Participant observation: _____

_____

_____

o. Sign system: _____

_____

_____

p. Time sampling: _____

_____

_____

q. Q sort: _____

_____

_____

r. Projective technique: _____

_____

_____

2. Below are several research problems. Indicate which type of unstructured self-report approach you might recommend using for each. Defend your response.

a. By what process do parents of a handicapped child learn to cope with their child's problem?

_____

_____

b. What are the barriers to preventive health care practices among the urban poor?

_____

_____

c. What stresses does the spouse of a terminally ill patient experience?

_____

_____

d. What types of information does a nurse draw on most heavily in formulating nursing diagnoses?

_____

_____

e. What are the health beliefs and health practices of elderly Native Americans living on a reservation?

_____

_____

3. Below are hypothetical responses of respondent Y and respondent Z to the Likert statements presented in Table 8-3 of the text. What would the total score for both of these respondents be, using the scoring rules described in Chapter 8?

Item No.	Respondent Y	Respondent Z
1	D	SA
2	A	D
3	SA	D
4	?	A
5	D	SA
6	SA	D
Total score:		

4. Below are hypothetical responses for respondents A, B, C, and D to the Likert statements presented in Table 8-3 of the text. Three of these four sets of responses contain some indication of a possible response set bias. Identify *which* three, and identify the types of bias.

Item No.	Respondent A	Respondent B	Respondent C	Respondent D
1	A	SA	SD	D
2	A	SD	SA	SD
3	SA	D	SA	D
4	A	A	SD	SD
5	?	A	SD	SD
7	A	D	SA	D
6	SA	SD	SA	D

5. Below are 10 attitudinal statements regarding attitudes toward natural family planning. For each statement, indicate how you think the item would be scored (*i.e.,* would "strongly agrees" be assigned a score of 1 or 5)? What are the maximum and minimum scores possible on this scale?

Statement	*Score for "Strongly Agree"*
a. Natural family planning is an effective method of avoiding unwanted pregnancies.	_____
b. Natural family planning removes the spontaneity from love making.	_____
c. Using natural family planning methods is too time-consuming.	_____
d. A man and a woman can be drawn closer together by collaborating in using natural family planning.	_____
e. Natural family planning is the safest form of birth control.	_____
f. Natural family planning is too risky if one really doesn't want a pregnancy.	_____
g. Natural family planning puts a woman in better touch with her body.	_____
h. Natural family planning is an acceptable form of contraception.	_____
i. All in all, natural family planning is the best method of birth control developed.	_____
j. Natural family planning is "unnatural" in terms of the restrictions it imposes on a couple's intimacy.	_____

6. Below are 10 problem statements in which the dependent variable of interest is amenable to observation. Specify whether you think a structured or unstructured approach would be preferable and justify your response. Also, consider the extent to which reactivity might be a problem during the collection of observational data and make a recommendation regarding the degree to which the researcher should be concealed.

a. What is the effect of touch on the crying behavior of hospitalized children?

_____

_____

b. What is the effect of increased patient/staff ratios in psychiatric hospitals on interpersonal conflict among staff members?

_____

_____

c. Is the management of appetite loss in burn patients affected by nutritional information provided by nurses?

_____

_____

d. Is the amount and type of information transmitted at the change-of-shift report affected by the number of years of experience of the nurses?

_____

_____

e. Does a patient's need for personal space vary as a function of age?

_____

_____

f. Are the self-grooming activities of nursing home patients related to the frequency of visits from friends and relatives?

_____

_____

g. Is the adequacy of a student nurse's handwashing related to his or her type of educational preparation?

_____

_____

h. What is the process by which very low-birth-weight infants develop the sucking response?

_____

_____

i. What type of patient behaviors are most likely to elicit empathic behaviors in nurses?

_____

_____

    j. Do nurses reinforce passive behaviors among female patients more than among male patients?

_____

_____

7. Below are five statements that might appear on Q-sort cards. For each, describe different continua according to which the cards could be sorted (*e.g.,* one continuum could be "very much like me/not at all like me" for a statement such as "I like to go to parties").

    a. Americans should be better educated with respect to nutrition.   _____

    b. Nursing students need to understand the fundamentals of research methods.   _____

    c. Insomnia   _____

    d. Good fringe benefits   _____

    e. A course on human sexual development   _____

8. Indicate which of the measures below is an in vivo measure and which is an in vitro measure:

    a. Blood pressure measures   _____

    b. Electrocardiogram measures   _____

    c. Hemoglobin concentration   _____

    d. Total lung capacity   _____

    e. Blood gas analysis of P_{CO_2} _____

    f. Chronoscope measures   _____

    g. Nasopharyngeal culture   _____

    h. Goniometer readings   _____

    i. Axillary temperature   _____

    j. Blood pH   _____

9. Three nurse researchers were collaborating on a study of the effect of visits to surgical patients preoperatively by operating room nurses on the stress levels of those patients just before surgery. One researcher wanted to use the patients' self-reports on a standardized scale to measure stress; the second suggested using pulse rate; the third recommended the patients' white blood cell count. Which measure do you feel would be the most appropriate for this research problem? Justify your response.

10. Identify five types of available records readily accessible to nurses that could be used to conduct a research study.

a. _____

_____

_____

b. _____

_____

_____

c. _____

_____

_____

d. _____

_____

_____

e. _____

_____

_____

▌ D. APPLICATION EXERCISES

1. Alongi (1993)* conducted a survey that focused on drug use patterns in an urban adolescent population. The survey used self-administered questionnaires that were distributed to 25 high schools and administered in group (home room) sessions to 3568 respondents. The questionnaire consisted of 56 closed-ended and two open-ended questions. Included were background questions; questions on the students' attitudes toward, knowledge of, and experience with various drugs; and questions on the students' physical and mental health. The instrument was pretested with 10 college freshmen before administration.

Review and critique the above description of the overall study. Suggest possible alternative ways of collecting the data for this study. To assist you in your critique, here are some guiding questions. (Review also the critiquing guidelines in Box 8-1 of the textbook.)

a. The data in this study were collected by self-report. Could the data have been collected in another way? *Should* they have been, in your opinion?

---

*This example is fictitious.

   b. Were the data collected by questionnaire or interview? Was the decision to use this method appropriate or would you recommend an alternative procedure? Comment on the advantages and disadvantages of the procedure used for this particular research problem.

   c. Comment on the degree of structure of the data collection approach. Would you recommend a more structured or a less structured approach? Why or why not?

   d. Were the instrument and procedures adequately pretested?

   e. Comment on the method in which the data were collected (*i.e.,* how was the instrument administered?). Was the method efficient? Did it yield an adequate response rate? Did it appear costly? What opportunity did respondents have to obtain clarifying information about the questions?

2. Below are several suggested research articles. Skim one of these articles, paying particular attention to the methods used to measure research variables and collect the data. Then respond to parts a to e of Question D.1 above in terms of this study.

   ■ Diaz, A. L., & McMillin, J. D. (1991). A definition and description of nurse abuse. *Western Journal of Nursing Research, 13,* 97–108.

   ■ Kearney, M. H., Cronenwett, L. R., & Barrett, J. A. (1990). Breast-feeding problems in the first week postpartum. *Nursing Research, 39,* 90–95.

   ■ Norberg, A., & Asplund, K. (1990). Caregivers' experience of caring for severely demented patients. *Western Journal of Nursing Research, 12,* 75–84.

   ■ Robb, H., Beltran, E. D., Katz, D., & Foxman, B. (1991). Sociodemographic factors associated with AIDS knowledge in a random sample of university students. *Public Health Nursing, 8,* 113–117.

   ■ Yonge, O. & Stewin, L. L. (1992). What psychiatric nurses say about constant care. *Clinical Nursing Research, 1,* 80–90.

3. Lovely (1992)† wanted to conduct a survey of nurses' attitudes toward abortion. For this study, she prepared 20 pro and con statements. After developing the items, she asked 10 of her colleagues to indicate their level of agreement or disagreement with the statements, on a seven-point scale. Lovely used the data from these 10 nurses as pretest data for refining the instrument. The original 20 items are presented below:

      1. Every woman has a right to obtain an abortion if she does not want a baby.

      2. Abortion should be made available to women on demand.

   *3. The government should subsidize the cost of abortions for poor women.

      4. Abortions should be made illegal.

      5. The right to an abortion should be available to all women.

---

†This example is fictitious.

*6. Women whose lives are in danger because of their pregnancy should be allowed to have an abortion.
  7. Abortion is morally wrong.
  8. Women need to have control of their own bodies by having abortion services available to them.
  9. Women who have abortions are murderers.
  10. People who oppose abortions have no compassion for women's circumstances.
  11. Legalizing abortion is a sign of the decay of civilization.
  12. No real woman would ever consider killing her own baby through abortion.
  13. The freedom to choose an abortion is essential to the liberation of women.
  14. An enlightened society gives its citizens the right to make important choices, such as having an abortion.
  15. The right to obtain a legal abortion should never be denied to women.
  16. Women who have abortions deserve praise for their courage to make a tough decision.
  17. No woman should be forced to bear a baby she does not want.
*18. If men had to bear babies, abortions would never have been illegal.
  19. Abortion is one of the most despicable acts that a human can commit.
  20. Having an abortion is better than having a child that would go unloved.

Upon reviewing the pretest responses, Lovely eliminated items 3, 6, and 18 (indicated with an asterisk). She then had a 17-item scale ready to use in her survey.

Read and critique the description of Lovely's activities. Suggest possible alternative ways of collecting the data for the research problem. To assist you in your critique, some guiding questions are presented below. (Review the critiquing guidelines in Box 8-2 of the textbook as well.)

a. What type of scale did the researcher develop? Was this type of scale best suited to the needs of the research, or would another type of scale have been more appropriate? Why or why not?
b. Given the aims of the researcher, was the development of *any* type of scale appropriate? That is, could the data have been collected by another method? *Should* they have been, in your opinion?
c. Comment on the procedures used by the researcher to develop the scale. Was the scale adequately reviewed and pretested?
d. Critique the quality of the scale itself. Does it consist of a sufficient number of items? Is the number of response alternatives good? Does the scale do an adequate job of minimizing bias? If not, suggest modifications that might reduce response set biases.

e. Comment on why you think the items that were eliminated (items 3, 6, and 18) were removed from the final scale.

f. Do you feel the researcher needed to develop this scale from scratch?

4. Below are several suggested research articles in which one or more scales were used. Review one of the articles and respond to parts a to f of Question D.3, to the extent possible, in terms of this study. (N.B.: The more technical aspects of the studies should just be briefly skimmed for the present exercise.)

   ▪ Bidigare, S. A., & Oermann, M. H. (1991). Attitudes and knowledge of nurses regarding organ procurement. *Heart and Lung, 20,* 20–24.

   ▪ Brown, M. S., & Tanner, C. (1990). Measurement of Type A behavior in preschoolers. *Nursing Research, 39,* 207–211.

   ▪ Forrester, D. A. (1990). AIDS-related risk factors, medical diagnosis, do-not-resuscitate orders and aggressiveness of nursing care. *Nursing Research, 39,* 350–354.

   ▪ Gulanick, M. (1991). Is Phase 2 cardiac rehabilitation necessary for early recovery of patients with cardiac disease? *Heart and Lung, 20,* 9–15.

5. Bingham (1993)‡ studied the effect of a school nutritional program on the snacking behaviors of students in grades 1 through 6. During the month of October, the experimental program (which consisted of discussion groups led by the school nurse, posters, and classroom activities initiated by the teachers) was introduced into two elementary schools in a large Eastern city. Two other schools were used as the controls. The children in all four schools were observed with respect to their selection of snack foods, offered once a week at a 2:00 PM "snack break." Each snack selected was rated in terms of its nutritional value on a scale from 1 to 9. The observations were made by the school nurses who were in the classrooms and noted the selection of each student. Similar observations were made during the months of October (when the program was implemented) and November (after the program was completed). The data consisted of two main types of information: (1) the frequency with which each snack item was selected each week, and (2) the nutritional ratings for the selected snacks for each child. An analysis of these data revealed that the children in the experimental classrooms selected significantly fewer snacks categorized as "nonnutritional salty snacks" (*e.g.,* potato chips) and had a significantly higher average nutritional rating in November than children in the comparison classrooms.

   Review and critique this study. Suggest alternative ways of collecting the data for the research problem. To assist you in your critique, here are some guiding questions. (Refer also to the questions in Box 8-3 of the textbook.)

---

‡This example is fictitious.

    a. The data in this study were collected by observation. Could the data have been collected in another way? *Should* they have been, in your opinion?

    b. Specify the relationship between the observer and those being observed in terms of the degree to which the observer was concealed. Do you feel that this relationship was appropriate? What kinds of problems might it create?

    c. Would you classify the study as having used an unstructured or structured observational procedure? Was the amount of structure in the data collection appropriate, or should there have been more or less structure?

    d. Was the specific procedure used to measure the study variables an adequate way to operationalize the variables? Could you recommend any improvements?

    e. What type of sampling plan was used to sample observations in this study? Would an alternative sampling plan have been better? Why or why not?

    f. What types of observational bias do you think might be operational in this study?

    g. Comment on the appropriateness of the people who made the observations. Can you identify any potential problems with respect to the internal and external validity of the study?

6. Below are several suggested research articles in which an observational approach was used. Review one of the articles and respond to parts a to g of Question D.5, to the extent possible, in terms of this study.

- Fegley, B. J. (1988). Preparing children for radiologic procedures: Contingent versus noncontingent instruction. *Research in Nursing and Health, 11,* 3–9.

- Harrison, M. J. (1990). A comparison of parental interactions with term and preterm infants. *Research in Nursing and Health, 13,* 173–179.

- Miller, D. B. & Holditch-Davis, D. (1992). Interactions of parents and nurses with high-risk preterm infants. *Research in Nursing & Health, 15,* 187–197.

- Swanson, K. M. (1991). Empirical development of a middle range theory of caring. *Nursing Research, 40,* 161–166.

- Yeomans, A., Davitt, M., Peters, C. A., Pastuszek, C., & Cobb, S. (1991). Efficacy of chlorhexidine gluconate use in the prevention of perirectal infections in patients with acute leukemia. *Oncology Nursing Forum, 18,* 1207–1212.

7. Malinowski (1993)[§] used a combination of projective techniques to study children's fears of hospitalization. Forty children were randomly assigned to an experimental or control condition. The experimental group received a special treatment designed to alleviate prehospitalization anxiety in school-

---

§This example is fictitious.

aged children. Controls did not receive any special instruction or treatment. The groups were then compared in terms of their responses to several projective measures, including the following:

- Responses to three cartoons that showed a hospitalized child interacting with hospital staff in three settings (as the child was being taken to the operating rooms; as the child was given medication; and as the child was eating). The children were asked to complete the dialogue by indicating the response of the hospitalized child.
- Sentence completions that included the following items: "I think nurses are...."; "Being in a hospital is..."; "I feel...."
- Play technique involving the use of dolls. Two dolls are given to the child, and the child is asked to play out a scene between a hospitalized child and a playmate, who comes to visit him or her in the hospital.

Read and critique the description of Malinowski's activities. Suggest possible alternative ways of collecting the data for the research problem. To assist you in your critique, here are some guiding questions.

a. Which of the methods described in Chapter 8 did the researcher employ? Was this a good selection? Would you recommend that the researcher switch to an alternative method, such as other methods described in Chapter 8? Why or why not?

b. Comment on the techniques used in terms of response set biases.

c. Comment on the techniques used in terms of the degree of objectivity of measuring the critical variables.

d. Comment on the techniques used in terms of the efficiency of the procedure (*i.e.*, amount of time required by subjects and researcher in regard to the amount of data yielded).

e. Comment on the techniques in terms of appropriateness for the study sample.

8. Below are three suggested research articles in which projective techniques were used. Review one of the articles and respond to parts a to e of Question D.7, to the extent possible, in terms of this study.

- Logsdon, D. A. (1991). Conceptions of health and health behaviors of preschool children. *Journal of Pediatric Nursing, 6,* 396–406.
- Spitzer, A. (1992). Children's knowledge of illness and treatment experiences in hemophilia. *Journal of Pediatric Nursing, 7,* 43–51.
- Walker, C. L. (1988). Stress and coping in siblings of childhood cancer patients. *Nursing Research, 37,* 208–212.

9. Van Vlieberghe (1992)[||] conducted a quasi-experimental study of the effectiveness of a program for treating the physiologic anemia associated with pregnancy. The experimental treatment involved instruction regarding a nu-

---

[||] This example is fictitious.

tritional regimen. The experimental group received verbal instructions by a nurse-midwife regarding dietary requirements and a list of foods known to be high in iron. Recommended daily amounts of certain foods were prescribed. The intervention also involved follow-up telephone conversations with the experimental group members at the 30th and 34th weeks of the pregnancy to discuss dietary and nutritional concerns. The comparison group members were given information that is normally given to pregnant women, with no individual follow-up. Fifty pregnant women who were outpatients at one hospital clinic served as the experimental subjects, and 50 pregnant women who were clients at an HMO served as the comparison group subjects. Van Vlieberghe chose hematocrit readings as the measure of effectiveness of the experimental intervention. During the 6th month of the pregnancy, and again at the 36th-week visit, a hematocrit laboratory test was performed. The data were analyzed by comparing the degree of change that had occurred in the two hematocrit readings within the two groups. The researcher found that there were no significant differences in physiologic anemia in the two groups, as measured by the changes in hematocrit tests.

Review and critique this study. Suggest alternative ways of collecting the data for the research problem. To assist you in your critique, here are some guiding questions. (Refer also to the questions in Box 8-4 of the textbook.)

   a. The data in this study were collected by a biophysiologic measure. Could the data have been collected in another way? In your opinion, should they have been?
   b. Is the measure used an in vivo or in vitro type of measurement? Is it an invasive or noninvasive type of procedure?
   c. Comment on the objectivity of the data collection method. How does its objectivity compare with other methods of measuring the dependent variable (*e.g.,* observations of pallor of the skin, mucous membranes, and fingernail beds)?
   d. What other biophysiologic measures might have been used to collect data in the study?

10. Below are several suggested research articles in which a biophysiologic measure was used. Review one of the articles and respond to parts a to d of Question D.9, to the extent possible, in terms of the study.

   ■ Janson-Bjerklie, S., Ferketich, S., Benner, P., & Becker, G. (1992). Clinical markers of asthma severity and risk: Importance of subjective as well as objective factors. *Heart & Lung, 21,* 265–272.
   ■ Levine-Silverman, S., & Johnson, J. (1990). Pulmonary artery pressure measurements. *Western Journal of Nursing Research, 12,* 488–496.
   ■ Westfall, U. E., & Heitkemper, M. M. (1992). Systemic responses to different enteral feeding schedules in rats. *Nursing Research, 41,* 144–150.

■ Yucha, C. B., Hastings-Tolsma, M., Szeverenyi, N. M., Tompkins, J. M., & Robson, L. (1991). Characterization of intravenous infiltrates. *Applied Nursing Research, 4,* 184–186.

▌ E. SPECIAL PROJECTS

1. Develop a topic guide for studying barriers to health-care utilization among the urban poor.
2. Suggest one open-ended and one closed-ended question relating to each of the following variables. Compare the quality and amount of information that could be obtained with each.
   a. Women's attitudes toward nurse-midwives
   b. Factors influencing a decision to obtain a vasectomy
   c. Perceived adequacy of community health care services
   d. Student nurses' first experiences with the death of a patient
   e. Factors influencing nurses' administration of pain-relieving narcotics to patients
3. Suppose that you were interested in studying hospitalized patients' satisfaction with their nursing care. Develop five positively worded and five negatively worded statements that could be used to construct a Likert scale for such a study.
4. Below is a list of five variables. Indicate briefly how you might operationalize each using structured observational procedures.
   a. Fear in hospitalized children
   b. Pain during childbirth
   c. Dependency in psychiatric patients
   d. Empathy in nursing students
   e. Cooperativeness in chemotherapy patients
5. Develop a problem statement for a study that could use observational data collection procedures. Make a recommendation regarding the use of a structured or unstructured approach for this problem.
6. Suppose that you wanted to evaluate the effect of an experimental nursing intervention on the well-being and comfort of cardiac patients. Indicate several physiologic measures you might consider using in such a study. Evaluate each of your suggestions with respect to ease of obtaining the data, relevance, and objectivity.
7. Using procedures described in Chapter 8, suggest methods of collecting data on the following: fear of death among the elderly; body image among amputees; reactions to the onset of menarche; nurses' morale in an emergency room; and dependence among cerebral-palsied children.

IIIIII Chapter 9
Data Quality

II A. MATCHING EXERCISES

1. Match each statement from Set B with one of the phrases from Set A. Indicate the letter corresponding to your response next to each of the statements in Set B.

Set A

a. Reliability
b. Validity
c. Both reliability and validity
d. Neither reliability nor validity

Set B   *Responses*

1. Is concerned with the accuracy of quantitative measures   _____
2. The measures must be high on this in order for the results of a quantitative study to be valid   _____
3. If a quantitative measure possesses this, it is necessarily valid   _____
4. Can in some cases be estimated by procedures that yield a quantified coefficient   _____
5. Can be enhanced by lengthening (adding subparts to) a scale   _____
6. Is necessarily high when the measure is high on objectivity   _____
7. Is concerned with whether the researcher has adequately conceptualized the variables under investigation   _____
8. Equivalence is one aspect of this   _____

2. Match each statement from Set B with one of the phrases from Set A. Indicate the letter corresponding to your response next to each of the statements in Set B.

Set A

a. Data triangulation
b. Investigator triangulation
c. Theory triangulation
d. Method triangulation

Set B   *Responses*

1. A researcher studying health beliefs of the rural elderly
   interviews old people and health care providers in the area.   _____

2. A researcher tests narrative data, collected in interviews with
   people who attempted suicide, against two alternative
   explanations of stress and coping.   _____

3. Two researchers independently interview 10 informants in a
   study of adjustment to a cancer diagnosis, and debrief with
   each other to review what they have learned.   _____

4. A researcher studying school-based clinics observes
   interactions in the clinics and also conducts in-depth
   interviews with students.   _____

5. A researcher studying the process of resolving an infertility
   problem interviews husbands and wives separately.   _____

6. Themes emerging in the field notes of an observer on a
   psychiatric ward are categorized and labeled independently by
   the researcher and an assistant.   _____

▌ B. COMPLETION EXERCISES

Write the words or phrases that correctly complete the sentences below.

1. People are not measured directly; their _____
   are measured.

2. The procedure known as _____ refers to
   the assignment of numeric information to indicate how much of an attribute is
   present.

3. In measurement, numbers are assigned according to specified _____
   _____ .

4. In theory, measurement involves _____
   from a hypothetical universe.

5. Obtained scores almost always consist of an error component and a _____
   _____ component.

6. From a measurement perspective, response set biases represent a source of
   _____ .

7. A reliable measure is one that maximizes the _____
   component of observed scores.

8. Test–retest reliability focuses on the _____
   of a measure.

9. The internal consistency of a measure can be assessed through a procedure known as the _____ technique, which involves dividing the items of an instrument into two parts.

10. Another term for internal consistency is _____ .

11. Procedures that examine the proportion of agreements between two independent judges yield estimates of _____ .

12. An instrument that is not reliable cannot be _____ .

13. The type of validity that focuses on the representativeness of the subparts of a measure is _____ validity.

14. The type of validity that deals with the ability of an instrument to distinguish people who differ in terms of some future criterion is _____ validity.

15. The four criteria for establishing the trustworthiness of qualitative data are _____ , _____ , _____ , and _____ .

16. When a qualitative researcher undertakes a _____ in the field, he or she has more opportunity to develop trust with informants and to test for possible misinformation.

17. The use of multiple sources of information in a study as a means of verification is known as _____ .

18. The technique of debriefing with informants to evaluate the credibility of qualitative data is referred to as _____ .

19. The criterion of _____ refers to the objectivity or neutrality of the data.

20. In qualitative studies, a(n) _____ of data and documents by an independent reviewer can verify the dependability and neutrality of the data and their interpretation.

▌ C. STUDY QUESTIONS

1. Define the following terms. Use the textbook to compare your definition with the definition in Chapter 9 or in the Glossary.

   a. Measurement: _____
   _____
   _____

b. Obtained score: _____

_____

_____

c. Error of measurement: _____

_____

_____

d. Reliability: _____

_____

_____

e. Test–retest reliability: _____

_____

_____

f. Reliability coefficient: _____

_____

_____

g. Internal consistency: _____

_____

_____

h. Split-half technique: _____

_____

_____

i. Cronbach's alpha: _____

_____

_____

j. Interrater reliability: _____

_____

_____

k. Validity: _____

_____

_____

l. Content validity: _____

_____

_____

m. Criterion-related validity: _____

_____

_____

n. Construct validity: _____

_____

_____

o. Known-groups technique: _____

_____

_____

p. Triangulation: _____

_____

_____

q. Transferability of data: _____

_____

_____

r. Audit trail: _____

_____

_____

s. Psychometric evaluation: _____

_____

_____

2. The reliability of measures of which of the following attributes would not be appropriately assessed using a test–retest procedure with 1 week between administrations? Why?

a. Attitudes toward abortion:

_____

_____

b. Stress:

_____

_____

c. Achievement motivation:

_____

_____

d. Nursing effectiveness:

_____

_____

e. Depression:

_____

_____

3. Comment on the meaning and implications of the following statement.

> *A researcher found that the internal consistency of her 20-item scale measuring attitudes toward nurse-midwives was .74, using the Cronbach alpha formula.*

4. In the situation described below, what might some of the sources of measurement error be?

> *A sample of 100 nurses who worked in a large metropolitan hospital were asked to complete a 10-item Likert scale designed to measure job satisfaction. The questionnaires were distributed by nursing supervisors at the end of shifts. The staff nurses were asked to complete the forms and return them immediately to their supervisors.*

5. Identify what is incorrect about the following statements:

a. "My scale is highly reliable, so it must be valid."

_____

_____

b. "My instrument yielded an internal consistency coefficient of .80, so it must be stable."

_____

_____

c. "The validity coefficient between my scale and a criterion measure was .40; therefore, my scale must be of low validity."

_____

_____

d. "The validation study proved that my measure has construct validity."

_____

_____

e. "My advisor examined my new measure of dependence in nursing home residents and, based on its content, assured me the measure was valid."

_____

_____

‖ D. APPLICATION EXERCISES

1. Rosen (1993)* wanted to study paternal bonding and attachment among men who had recently become fathers. Her main objective was to compare paternal attachment among men who had participated with their wives in prenatal classes and were present during childbirth with men who had not. In reviewing prior work in this area, Rosen was unable to identify a paternal attachment scale that she found suitable to her needs. Therefore, she developed her own scale to measure paternal attachment. Her scale consisted of 10 statements that respondents were asked to rate as "very much like me," "somewhat like me," or "not at all like me." An example of the statements on the scale is: "The birth of my baby aroused sentiments of immediate affection, closeness, and pride." Total scores were obtained by using procedures analogous to those used for summated rating scales.

Rosen pretested her scale with 30 men within 48 hours of the delivery of their babies. The internal consistency of the scale was assessed using the split-half technique, which yielded a reliability coefficient of .68. In terms of validating the instrument, Rosen used two approaches. First, she invited two colleagues who worked in maternal-child nursing to review the 10 statements and evaluate them in terms of content validity. Second, she asked nurses who worked in the hospital maternity ward to provide ratings, on a 0-to-10 scale, of how attached each new father appeared to be, based on the nurses' observations of the fathers' behavior in regard to their babies. The correlations between the fathers' scale scores and the nurses' ratings was .56.

Review and critique this research effort. Suggest alternative ways of assessing the quality of the data collection instrument. To assist you in your critique, answer the guiding questions below. (Refer also to the relevant critiquing guidelines in Box 9-1 of the textbook.)

a. What method was used to assess the reliability of the instrument? On what aspect of reliability does this method focus? Is this focus appropriate? Should some alternative method for estimating reliability have been used? Should an _additional_ method of estimating reliability have been used?

_____

*This example is fictitious.

    b. Comment on the adequacy of the instrument's reliability. Should the reliability be better? If so, what might the researcher do to improve the reliability?

    c. What method was used to assess the validity of the instrument? On what aspect of validity does this approach focus? Is this focus appropriate? Should some alternative method for estimating validity have been used? Should an *additional* method of estimating validity have been used?

    d. Comment on the adequacy of the instrument's validity. Should the validity be better? If so, what might the researcher do to improve the validity?

2. Below are several suggested research articles. Read one of these articles, paying special attention to the ways the researcher assessed the adequacy of his or her measuring tool. Evaluate the measurement strategy, using parts a to d of Question D.1 as a guide. (Ignore the more technical aspects of the report, such as those that deal with factor analysis.)

- Clough, D. H. (1991). The effects of cognitive distortion and depression on disability in rheumatoid arthritis. *Research in Nursing and Health, 14,* 439–446.
- Fortier, J. C., Carson, V. B., Will, S., & Shubkagel, B. L. (1991). Adjustment to a newborn: Sibling preparation makes a difference. *Journal of Obstetric, Gynecologic, and Neonatal Nursing, 20,* 73–79.
- Murphy, P. A., Forrester, D. A., Price, D. M., & Monaghan, J. F. (1992). Empathy of intensive care nurses and critical care family needs assessment. *Heart and Lung, 21,* 25–30.
- Tompkins, E. S. (1992). Nurse/client values congruence. *Western Journal of Nursing Research, 14,* 225–236.

3. Below are several suggested research reports on qualitative studies. Read one of the articles, paying special attention to the ways in which the researcher addressed data quality issues. Use the relevant guidelines in Box 9-1 to assist you in your appraisal of the data's trustworthiness and the researcher's efforts to document it.

- Beck, C. T. (1992). The lived experience of postpartum depression: A phenomenological study. *Nursing Research, 41,* 166–170.
- Bright, M. A. (1992). Making place: The first birth in an intergenerational family context. *Qualitative Health Research, 2,* 75–98.
- Fleury, J. D. (1991). Empowering potential: A theory of wellness motivation. *Nursing Research, 40,* 286–291.
- Keller, C. (1991). Seeking normalcy: The experience of coronary artery bypass surgery. *Research in Nursing and Health, 14,* 173–178.

▌ E. SPECIAL PROJECTS

1. Develop a problem statement (or a hypothesis) for a nursing research study that would require a quantitative data collection approach. Prepare operational definitions that specify measurement rules for the variables in your statement.

2. Suppose that you were developing an instrument to measure attitudes toward test-tube babies. Your measure consists of 15 Likert-type items. Describe what you would do to (a) estimate the reliability of your scale and (b) assess the validity of your scale.

3. Suggest the type of groups that might be used to validate measures of the following concepts using the known-groups technique:
   a. Self-esteem
   b. Empathy
   c. Capacity for self-care
   d. Emotional dependence
   e. Depression

4. Suppose you were interested in conducting an in-depth study of women who had been raped. Describe ways in which you might achieve (a) data triangulation, (b) method triangulation, (c) member checks.

Analysis of Research Data

Part V

||||||| Chapter 10
Quantitative Analysis

▌ A. MATCHING EXERCISES

1. Match each variable in Set B with the level of measurement from Set A that captures the highest possible level for that variable. Indicate the letter corresponding to your response next to each variable in Set B.

Set A

a. Nominal scale
b. Ordinal scale

c. Interval scale
d. Ratio scale

Set B   *Responses*

1. Hours spent in labor before childbirth   _____
2. Religious affiliation   _____
3. Time to first postoperative voiding   _____
4. Responses to a single Likert scale item   _____
5. Temperature on the centigrade scale   _____
6. Nursing specialty area   _____
7. Status on the following scale: in poor health; in fair health; in good health; in excellent health   _____
8. Pulse rate   _____
9. Score on a 25-item Likert scale   _____
10. Highest college degree attained (bachelor's, master's, doctorate)   _____
11. Apgar scores   _____
12. Membership in the American Nurses' Association   _____

2. Match each statement or phrase from Set B with one of the phrases from Set A. Indicate the letter corresponding to your response next to each of the statements in Set B.

Set A

a. Measure(s) of central tendency
b. Measure(s) of variability
c. Measure(s) of neither central tendency nor variability
d. Measure(s) of both central tendency and variability

Set B   *Responses*

1. The range   _____
2. In lay terms, an average   _____
3. A percentage   _____
4. A parametric statistic   _____
5. Descriptor(s) of a distribution of scores   _____
6. Descriptor(s) of how heterogeneous a set of values is   _____
7. The standard deviation   _____
8. The mode   _____
9. Is normally positively skewed   _____
10. The median   _____

3. Match each phrase or statement from Set B with one of the phrases in Set A. Indicate the letter corresponding to your response next to each of the statements in Set B.

Set A

a. Parametric test
b. Nonparametric test
c. Neither parametric nor nonparametric tests
d. Both parametric and nonparametric tests

Set B   *Responses*

1. The chi-squared test   _____
2. Paired t-test   _____
3. Researcher establishes the risk of Type I errors   _____
4. Used when a score distribution is nonnormal   _____
5. Offers proof that the null hypothesis is either true or false   _____
6. Assumes the dependent variable is measured on an interval or
   ratio scale   _____
7. Uses sample data to estimate population values   _____
8. ANOVA F-ratio   _____
9. Computed statistics are compared to tabled values based on
   theoretical distributions   _____
10. Used when there is only one variable   _____

4. Match each phrase from Set B with one (or more) of the statistical analyses presented in Set A. Indicate the letter corresponding to your response next to each of the statements in Set B.

Set A

a. Multiple regression analysis
b. Discriminant function analysis
c. Factor analysis
d. Logistic regression
e. Multivariate analysis of variance

Set B   *Responses*

1. Has more than one independent variable   _____
2. Yields an R^2 statistic   _____
3. Used to reduce variables to a smaller number of dimensions   _____
4. Has more than one dependent variable   _____
5. Is a multivariate statistical procedure   _____
6. Involves a dependent variable that is categorical (nominal level)   _____
7. Translates the probability of an event occurring into an odds ratio   _____
8. Is sometimes called MANOVA   _____

▌ B. COMPLETION EXERCISES

Write the words or phrases that correctly complete the sentence below.

1. Nominal measurement involves a simple _____ of objects according to some criterion.

2. Rank-order questions are an example of _____ measures.

3. With ratio-level measures there is a real, rational _____ .

4. Unlike ordinal measures, interval measures involve _____ between points on the scale.

5. A descriptive index (*e.g.,* percentage) from a population is called a(n) _____ _____ .

6. A(n) _____ is a systematic arrangement of quantitative data from lowest to highest values.

7. The symbol n represents the total _____ .

8. _____ are a common way of presenting frequency information in graphic form.

9. A distribution is described as _____ if the two halves are *mirror* images of each other.

10. A distribution is described as _____ skewed if its longer tail points to the left.

11. A distribution that has only one peak is said to be _____.

12. Many human characteristics, such as height and intelligence, are distributed to approximate a(n) _____.

13. Measures that summarize the typical value in a distribution are known as measures of _____.

14. Measures of _____ are concerned with how spread out the data are.

15. When scores are not very spread out (*i.e.*, dispersed over a wide range of values), the sample is said to be _____ with respect to that variable.

16. Descriptive statistics for two variables examined simultaneously are called _____.

17. Relationships are described as _____ if high values on one variable are associated with low values on a second.

18. The most commonly used correlation index is _____.

19. Researchers using quantitative analysis apply _____ to draw conclusions about a population based on information from a sample.

20. Sampling distributions of means have a _____ distribution.

21. The degree of risk of making a _____ error is controlled by the researcher.

22. Tests that involve the estimation of parameters are referred to as _____ tests.

23. The most commonly used _____ are the .05 and .01 levels.

24. Using $\alpha = .01$ rather than $\alpha = .05$ level *increases* the risk of committing a _____ error.

25. The statistic computed in an analysis of variance is the _____ statistic.

26. When both the independent and dependent variables are nominal measures, the test statistic usually calculated is the _____.

27. The square of _____ indicates the proportion of variance accounted for in a dependent variable by several independent variables.

28. ANCOVA is shorthand for _____.

29. In ANCOVA, the extraneous variable being controlled is referred to as the

    _____ .

30. In factor analysis, the underlying dimensions of a large set of variables are referred to as _____ .

31. The first phase in factor analysis is the _____ phase, in which the original variables are condensed into a smaller number of factors.

32. MANOVA is the acronym for _____ .

▌ C. STUDY QUESTIONS

1. Define the following terms. Use the textbook to compare your definition with the definition in Chapter 10 or in the Glossary.

   a. Level of measurement: _____

   _____

   _____

   b. Statistic: _____

   _____

   _____

   c. Skewed distribution: _____

   _____

   _____

   d. Bimodal distribution: _____

   _____

   _____

   e. Normal distribution: _____

   _____

   _____

   f. Median: _____

   _____

   _____

   g. Mean: _____

   _____

   _____

   h. Standard deviation: _____

   _____

   _____

i. Correlation coefficient: _____

_____

j. Sampling error: _____

_____

k. Sampling distribution: _____

_____

l. Standard error of the mean: _____

_____

m. Type I error: _____

_____

n. Type II error: _____

_____

o. Level of significance: _____

_____

p. Statistical significance: _____

_____

q. Nonparametric tests: _____

_____

r. *t*-test: _____

_____

s. Analysis of variance: _____

_____

t. Chi-squared test: _____

_____

   u. Multivariate statistics: _____

_____

   v. Multiple regression analysis: _____

_____

   w. Analysis of covariance: _____

_____

   x. Factor analysis: _____

_____

   y. Discriminant function analysis: _____

_____

   z. Logistic regression: _____

_____

2. Name five physiologic measures that yield ratio-level measurements.

   a. _____

   b. _____

   c. _____

   d. _____

   e. _____

3. Prepare a frequency distribution and frequency polygon for the set of scores below, which represent the ages of 30 women receiving estrogen replacement therapy:

47 50 51 50 48 51 50 51 49 51
54 49 49 53 51 52 51 52 50 53
49 51 52 51 50 55 48 54 53 52

    Describe the resulting distribution in terms of its symmetry and modality (*i.e.*, whether it is unimodal or multimodal).

4. Calculate the mean, median, and mode for the following pulse rates:

78 84 69 98 102 72 87 75 79 84 88 84 83 71 73

Mean: _____

Median: _____

Mode: _____

5. A group of nurse researchers measured the amount of time (in minutes) spent in recreational activities by a sample of 200 hospitalized paraplegic patients. They compared male and female patients as well as those aged 50 and younger versus those over 50 years old. The four group means (50 subjects per group) were as follows:

Age	Male	Female
≤50 years	98.2	70.1
>50 years	50.8	68.3

A two-way ANOVA yielded the following results:

	F	df	p
Sex	3.61	1,196	NS
Age group	5.87	1,196	<.05
Sex × Age group	6.96	1,196	<.01

Interpret the meaning of these results.

6. The correlation between the number of days absent per year and annual salary in a sample of 100 employees of an insurance company was found to be $-.23$ ($p < .05$). Discuss this result in terms of its meaning.

7. Indicate which statistical tests you would use to analyze data for the following variables:

a. Variable 1 is psychiatric patients' gender; variable 2 is whether or not the patient has attempted suicide in the past 6 months.

_____

_____

b. Variable 1 is the participation versus nonparticipation of patients with a pulmonary embolus in a special treatment group; variable 2 is the pH of the patients' arterial blood gases.

_____

_____

c. Variable 1 is serum creatinine concentration levels; variable 2 is daily urine output.

_____

_____

d. Variable 1 is patients' marital status (married versus divorced/separated/widowed versus never married); variable 2 is the patients' degree of self-reported depression (measured on a 30-item depression scale).

_____

_____

8. Suggest possible covariates that could be used to control extraneous variation in the following analyses:

a. An analysis of the effect of family income on the incidence of child abuse:

_____

_____

b. An analysis of the effect of age on patients' acceptance of pastoral counseling:

_____

_____

c. An analysis of the effect of therapeutic touch on patients' acceptance of pastoral counseling:

_____

_____

d. An analysis of the effect of need for achievement on students' attrition from a nursing program:

_____

_____

e. An analysis of the effect of faculty rank on faculty members' satisfaction with communications among colleagues:

_____

_____

9. In the following examples, which multivariate procedure is most appropriate for analyzing the data?

a. A researcher is testing the effect of verbal expressiveness, self-esteem, age, and the availability of family supports among a group of recently discharged psychiatric patients on recidivism (*i.e.*, whether they will be readmitted within 12 months after discharge).

_____

_____

b. A researcher is comparing the bereavement and coping processes of recently widowed and divorced individuals, controlling for their age.

_____

_____

c. A researcher wants to test the effects of two drug treatments and two dosages of each drug on blood pressure, and the pH and Po_2 levels of arterial blood gases.

_____

_____

d. A researcher wants to predict hospital staff absentee rates based on month of the year, staff rank, shift, number of years with the hospital, and marital status.

_____

_____

10. Below is a list of variables that a nurse researcher might be interested in predicting. For each, suggest at least three independent variables that could be used in a multiple regression analysis.

a. Leadership in nursing supervisors: _____

_____

b. Nurses' frequency of administering pain medication: _____

_____

c. Proficiency in doing patient interviews: _____

_____

d. Patient satisfaction with nursing care: _____

_____

e. Anxiety levels of prostatectomy patients: _____

_____

∥ D. APPLICATION EXERCISES

1. Bentley (1992)* hypothesized that infants' sleeping problems were related to various conditions and experiences during their birth. Fifty infants aged 3 to 6 months were diagnosed as having severe sleep-disturbance problems. A group of 50 infants aged 3 to 6 months who had normal sleeping patterns was used as the comparison group. Bentley obtained the hospital records for all 100 children. The two groups were compared in terms of the following variables: amount of anesthesia administered during labor and delivery (none, small amount, large amount); length of time in labor (number of hours and minutes); type of delivery (cesarean or vaginal); birth weight (in grams); and Apgar scores at 3 minutes (scores from 1 to 10). Bentley found that the sleep-disturbance group had had significantly longer time in labor than the comparison group. The groups were comparable in terms of the other variables.

   Review and critique this research effort. Suggest alternative measurement approaches. To assist you in your critique, here are some guiding questions.
   a. How many variables were measured in this study?
   b. For each variable, identify the level of measurement that was used.
   c. For each variable, indicate whether the measurement could have been made at a higher level of measurement than the level that was used. If yes, specify how you might measure the variable to obtain a higher level measure.
   d. For two of the variables, write out operational definitions that clearly indicate the rules of measurement for those variables.

2. Below are several suggested research articles. Read one of these articles, paying special attention to the ways in which the research variables were operationalized. Evaluate the researcher's measurement strategy, using parts **a** to **d** of Question D.1 as a guide.
   - Alexander, D., Gammage, D., Nichols, A., & Gaskins, D. (1992). Analysis of strike-through contamination in saturated sterile dressings. *Clinical Nursing Research, 1,* 28–34.
   - Cilenti, D., & Farel, A. M. (1991). Identifying infants at risk: North Carolina's high-priority infant program. *Public Health Nursing, 8,* 219–225.
   - Glenn, P. S. F., Nance-Spronson, L. E., McCartney, M., & Yesalis, C. E. (1991). Attitudes toward AIDS among a low-risk group of women. *Journal of Obstetric, Gynecologic, and Neonatal Nursing, 20,* 398–405.
   - Unkle, D., Smejkal, R., Snyder, R., Lessig, M., & Ross, S. E. (1991). Blood antibodies and uncrossmatched type O blood. *Heart and Lung, 20,* 284–286.

---

*This example is fictitious.

3. Langevin (1993)* hypothesized that patients with a high degree of physical mobility would describe themselves as being healthier than patients with less physical mobility. To test this hypothesis, 120 male patients in a Veterans Administration hospital were asked to rate themselves on a five-point scale regarding their current physical health (1 = very unhealthy and 5 = very healthy) and to predict the number of days that they would be hospitalized. Forty of these patients had been categorized as "of limited mobility," another 40 were classified as "of moderate mobility," and the remaining 40 were described as "of high mobility." Langevin reported his descriptive findings as follows:

> *The self-ratings of physical health were fairly normally distributed for the sample as a whole: 42% rated themselves as neither healthy nor unhealthy; 7% and 21% described themselves as "very healthy" or "somewhat healthy," respectively. At the other extreme, 6% said they were "very unhealthy," and 24% said "somewhat unhealthy." The three groups differed in this regard, however. In the high-mobility group, a full 45% said they were either "very" or "somewhat healthy," while only 30% of the moderate-mobility and 15% of the low-mobility groups said this.*

> *For the entire sample, the mean predicted length of stay was 14.1 days. The median length, however, was only 12.5 days. For the three groups, the means and standard deviations with respect to predicted length of stay in hospital were as follows:*

	Mean	Standard Deviation
High Mobility	7.1	3.2
Moderate Mobility	11.9	4.5
Low Mobility	23.3	7.4

> *In this sample of patients, the correlation between predicted length of stay in hospital and the health rating was .56.*

Review and critique this study, particularly with respect to the statistical analysis. To assist you in this critique, here are some guiding questions.

a. Was the mode of data analysis (*i.e.*, quantitative versus qualitative) appropriate? Why or why not?

---

*This example is fictitious.

b. Which of the following types of descriptive statistical methods were used in this example?
  - Frequency distribution
  - Measure of central tendency
  - Measure of variability
  - Contingency table
  - Correlation

c. Comment on the appropriateness of each statistic reported in the example. Is the statistic appropriate given the level of measurement of the variable? Does the statistic throw away information? Is the statistic the most stable statistic possible?

d. Identify two or three statistics that were not reported by the researcher that could have been reported given the data that were collected. Evaluate the extent to which the absence of this information weakened (or streamlined) the report of the results.

e. Discuss the meaning of the means and standard deviations in this example.

4. Below are several suggested research articles. Skim one (or more) of these articles and respond to parts **a** to **e** of Question D.3 in terms of the actual research study. (At this point, ignore the references to tests of statistical significance, which are covered in subsequent exercises.)

  - Andrews, C. M., & Chrzanowski, M. (1990). Maternal position, labor, and comfort. *Applied Nursing Research, 3,* 7–13.
  - Gardner, D. L. (1992). Conflict and retention of new graduate nurses. *Western Journal of Nursing Research, 14,* 76–85.
  - Hogan, N. S., & Balk, D. E. (1990). Adolescent reactions to sibling death: Perceptions of mothers, fathers, and teenagers. *Nursing Research, 39,* 103–106.
  - McFarlande, J., Christoffel, K., Bateman, L., Miller, V., & Bullock, L. (1991). Assessing for abuse: Self-report versus nurse interview. *Public Health Nursing, 8,* 245–250.
  - Primomo, J., Yates, B. C., & Woods, N. F. (1990). Social support for women during chronic illness. *Research in Nursing and Health, 13,* 153–161.

5. Kuhara (1992)* investigated whether taste acuity declines with age, using a cross-sectional design. Eighty subjects were given a taste acuity test in which they were asked to indicate, for 25 substances, whether the taste was salty, sweet, bitter, or sour. The substances were presented in randomized order. Each person had five scores: four scores corresponding to the correct identification of the substances in the four taste categories, and one total score. Twenty subjects from each of the following age groups were tested: 31 to 40; 41 to 50; 51 to 60; and 61 to 70 years. It was hypothesized that taste acuity would decline with age, both overall and for all four subcategories of taste.

---

*This example is fictitious.

The mean test scores for the four groups on all five outcomes measures appear below, together with information on the statistical tests performed.

	Age Group						
	31–40	*41–50*	*51–60*	*61–70*	*F*	*df*	*p*
Salty test	6.3	5.8	5.7	5.4	3.5	3,76	<.05
Sweet test	5.0	5.0	5.4	5.2	1.2	3,76	>.05
Bitter test	4.0	4.1	3.7	3.3	2.6	3,76	>.05
Sour test	1.9	2.0	2.0	2.1	0.8	3,76	>.05
Overall test	17.2	16.9	16.8	16.0	2.4	3,76	>.05

Kuhara concluded that her hypothesis was only partially supported by the data.

Review and critique the above study. Suggest possible alternatives for handling the analysis of the data. To assist you in your critique, here are some guiding questions.

a. For each of the variables, indicate the actual level of measurement as used, then indicate the highest possible level of measurement for each. Is there a discrepancy? If so, can you think of a justification for it?

b. What statistical test was used to analyze the data? Did the researcher use the appropriate statistical test? If not, what statistical test do you think would be more suitable?

c. Are the degrees of freedom as presented correct?

d. Which of the results is statistically significant—that is, which hypothesis was supported by the data? Describe the meaning of each of the statistical tests.

6. Below are several suggested research articles. Skim one (or more) of these articles and respond to parts **a** to **d** of Question D.5 in terms of the actual research study.

- Chen, S. C., Fitzgerald, M. C., DeStefano, L. M., & Chen, E. H. (1991). Effects of a school nurse prenatal counseling program. *Public Health Nursing, 8,* 212–218.

- Erickson, R. S., & Yount, S. T. (1991). Effect of aluminized covers on body temperature in patients having abdominal surgery. *Heart & Lung, 20,* 255–264.

- Kearney, M. H., & Cronenwett, L. (1991). Breastfeeding and employment. *Journal of Obstetric, Gynecologic, and Neonatal Nursing, 20,* 471–480.

- Miller, K. M., & Perry, P. A. (1990). Relaxation technique and postoperative pain in patients undergoing cardiac surgery. *Heart and Lung, 19,* 136–146.

- Shivnan, J. C., McGuire, D., Freedman, S., Sharkazy, E., Bosserman, G., Larson, E., & Grouleff, P. (1991). A comparison of transparent adherent and dry sterile gauze dressings for long-term central catheters in patients undergoing bone marrow transplant. *Oncology Nursing Forum, 18,* 1349–1356.

▌ E. SPECIAL PROJECTS

1. Fictitious data from 24 nurses for six variables are presented below. Compute and present 5 to 10 different descriptive statistics that you think would best summarize this information.

Subject No.	Shift[a]	Anxiety Scores[b]	Supervisor's Performance Rating[c]	No. of Years of Experience	Marital Status[d]	Job Satisfaction Score[e]
1	1	10	4	5	2	4
2	1	13	4	2	2	5
3	1	8	2	1	1	3
4	1	4	7	10	1	3
5	1	6	9	12	1	4
6	1	9	8	7	1	2
7	1	12	6	8	2	4
8	1	5	4	2	1	5
9	2	10	5	4	2	1
10	2	14	6	1	2	4
11	2	8	5	3	1	5
12	2	15	8	2	2	2
13	2	11	8	7	2	3
14	2	14	7	9	1	1
15	2	1	5	3	2	2
16	2	8	8	6	1	3
17	3	3	7	19	2	4
18	3	7	4	7	1	1
19	3	19	5	1	2	2
20	3	5	6	11	1	1
21	3	8	3	2	1	3
22	3	10	4	5	2	2
23	3	13	6	6	2	1
24	3	14	5	3	1	2

[a]1 = day; 2 = evening; 3 = night

[b]Scores are from a low of 0 to a high of 20, 20 = most anxious

[c]Ratings are from 1 = poor to 9 = excellent

[d]1 = married; 2 = not married

[e]Scores are from low of 1 to high of 5; 5 = most satisfied

2. Ask 20 friends, classmates, or colleagues the following three questions:
   - How many brothers and sisters do you have?
   - How many children do you expect to have in total?
   - Would you describe your family during your childhood as "very close," "fairly close," or "not very close"?

   When you have gathered your data, calculate and present several statistics that describe the information you obtained.

3. Below is a list of variables. Assume that you have data from 500 nurses on these variables. Develop two or three hypotheses regarding the relationships among these variables and indicate what statistical tests you would use to test your hypotheses.
   - Number of years of nursing experience
   - Type of employment setting (hospital, nursing school, public school system, etc.)
   - Salary
   - Marital status
   - Job satisfaction ("dissatisfied," "neither dissatisfied nor satisfied," or "satisfied")
   - Number of children under age 18
   - Gender

4. Design and describe a study in which you would use both factor analysis and discriminant function analysis.

IIIIIII Chapter 11
Qualitative Research and Analysis

II A. MATCHING EXERCISES

1. Match each descriptive statement from Set B with one of the statements from Set A. Indicate the letter corresponding to your response next to each item in Set B.

Set A
a. Qualitative data
b. Quantitative data
c. Both qualitative and quantitative data
d. Neither qualitative nor quantitative data

Set B   *Responses*

 1. Should be collected to help improve nursing practice   _____
 2. Are especially useful for understanding dynamic processes   _____
 3. Are often collected in large-scale surveys   _____
 4. Are useful in proving the validity of theories   _____
 5. Are usually collected by phenomenologic researchers   _____
 6. Can profit from triangulation   _____
 7. Are often used in tests of causal relationships   _____
 8. Can contribute to theoretical insights   _____
 9. Require validity checks   _____
10. Tend to be collected from small samples   _____

II B. COMPLETION EXERCISES

Write the words or phrases that correctly complete the sentences below.

1. The term *holistic* is more often used to describe _____ than _____ research.

2. In qualitative research, hypothesis _____ is frequently a goal.

3. Ethnographic research focuses on human _____.

4. Phenomenologic research focuses on the _____ of phenomena as experienced by people.

5. The disciplinary roots of ethnography is _____; of phenomenology is _____; and of ethno-methodology is _____.

6. The main task in organizing qualitative data involves the development of a method of _____ the data.

7. In developing conceptual files, the researcher must devise a comprehensive _____ scheme.

8. The analysis of qualitative data generally begins with a search for _____
_____.

9. The use of _____ involves an accounting of the frequency with which certain themes and relationships are supported by the data.

10. The approach known as _____ involves a constant comparative approach to collecting and analyzing qualitative data, with an eye toward theory development.

11. Qualitative and quantitative data are often _____ in that they mutually supply each other's lack.

12. A major advantage of integrating different approaches is potential enhance-ments to the study's _____.

▌ C. STUDY QUESTIONS

1. Define the following terms. Use the textbook to compare your definition with the definition in Chapter 11 or in the Glossary.

a. Qualitative analysis: _____
_____
_____

b. Emic perspective: _____
_____
_____

c. Etic perspective: _____
_____
_____

d. Ethnonursing research: _____

_____

_____

e. Bracketing: _____

_____

_____

f. Induction: _____

_____

_____

g. Grounded theory: _____

_____

_____

h. Saturation: _____

_____

_____

i. Multimethod research: _____

_____

_____

j. Content analysis: _____

_____

_____

2. For each of the problem statements below, indicate whether you think a researcher should collect primarily qualitative or quantitative data.

a. How do victims of AIDS cope with the discovery of their illness?

_____

_____

b. What important dimensions of nursing practice differ in developed and underdeveloped countries?

_____

_____

c. What is the effect of therapeutic touch on patient well-being?

_____

_____

d. Do nurse practitioners and physicians differ in the performance of triage functions?

_____

_____

e. Is a patient's length of stay in hospital related to the quality or quantity of his or her social supports?

_____

_____

f. How does the typical American feel about such new reproductive technologies as in vitro fertilization?

_____

_____

g. By what processes do women make decisions about having an amniocentesis?

_____

_____

h. What are the psychological sequelae of having an organ transplant?

_____

_____

i. What factors are most predictive of a woman giving birth to a very low-birth-weight infant?

_____

_____

j. What effects does caffeine have on gastrointestinal motility?

_____

_____

3. Read one of the following studies, in which qualitative data were gathered and analyzed to address a research question. Suggest ways in which the collection of quantitative data might have enriched the study, strengthened its validity, or enhanced its interpretability.
   - Blenner, J. L. (1990). Attaining self-care in infertility treatment. *Applied Nursing Research, 3,* 98–104.
   - Chapman, L. L. (1992). Expectant fathers' roles during labor and birth. *Journal of Obstetric, Gynecologic, and Neonatal Nursing, 21,* 114–120.
   - Mayo, K. (1992). Physical activity practices among American black working women. *Qualitative Health Research, 2,* 318–333.
   - VanDongen, C. J. (1990). Agonizing questioning: Experiences of survivors of suicide victims. *Nursing Research, 39,* 224–229.

4. Read one of the following studies, in which quantitative data were gathered and analyzed to address a research question. Suggest ways in which the collection of qualitative data might have enriched the study, strengthened its validity, or enhanced its interpretability.

- Froman, R. D., & Owen, S. V. (1990). Mothers' and nurses' perceptions of infant care skills. *Research in Nursing and Health, 13,* 247–253.
- Hicks, F. D., Larson, J. L., & Ferrans, C. E. (1992). Quality of life after liver transplant. *Research in Nursing and Health, 15,* 111–119.
- Walcott-McQuigg, J. A., & Ervin, N. E. (1992). Stressors in the workplace: Community health nurses. *Public Health Nursing, 9,* 65–70.
- White, N. E., Richter, J. M., & Fry, C. (1992). Coping, social support, and adaptation to chronic illness. *Western Journal of Nursing Research, 14,* 211–224.

▌ D. APPLICATION EXERCISES

1. Arpei (1993)* studied the phenomenon of "being on precautions" from the perspective of hospitalized adults. She began her study by spending 2 days on the hospital units where the data would be collected. The 2 days were spent familiarizing herself with the units, learning how best to collect the data, determining where she could position herself in an unobtrusive manner, and establishing a trusting relationship with the nursing staff.

The data for the study were collected using the techniques of observation and unstructured interviewing. Arpei selectively sampled all times of the day and all days of the week in 2-hour segments to make her observations. The time schedule began on a Monday morning at 7 AM and continued until 9 AM. On Tuesday, the observation time became 9 AM until 11 AM. Observations continued around the clock on consecutive days until no new information was being collected. Arpei positioned herself either directly outside the door to the patient's room or sat in the patient's room to make her observations. Observations included any activity or interaction between the patient and hospital staff or between the patient and herself.

The unstructured interviewing process consisted of asking patients to clarify why they were doing certain things and what they liked or disliked about the hospital experience.

Arpei recorded the observations and data from the interviews in a log immediately after each 2-hour observation segment. All data were recorded in chronologic order. In addition to the above, Arpei also recorded any feelings she had during the observation experience. As time progressed, she reread her field notes after every 4 hours of observation. As commonalities began to emerge from the data, she developed another section to her log according to similarity of content and referenced the daily log notes according to commonalities. Arpei continued making observations until she felt she had a "feel for

---

*This example is fictitious.

the data" and additional observations or interactions provided only redundant information. A total of four patients were observed.

Themes that emerged from the data were labeled "avoidance," "devaluation as a person," and "loneliness." Evidence for the avoidance perspective came from patient comments during informal conversations with the researcher and the observational field notes. The evidence included statements such as, "Nurses seldom come into the room because they have to put all that (pointing to precaution gowns) stuff on"; "Look, she (the cleaning woman) won't come in the room. She's afraid of me"; "Did you see that? Only my doctor would touch me. The rest were afraid to touch me." Observational field notes contained several notations of nurses coming to the door of the room asking, "Do you want anything?" but not entering the room.

The theme "loneliness" was developed from observations of patients occasionally putting the call light on to find out what time it was or how long until lunch, or asking about a noise they had heard. Comments that conveyed the same feeling of loneliness were "Being confined in this room is like being in jail"; "I can't wait to get out of here and have dinner with my friends"; and "The hours seem endless here."

Review and critique this study. Suggest alternative ways of collecting and analyzing the data for the research problem. To assist you in your critique, consider the following guiding questions, as well as the questions in Box 11-1 of the text.

a. Comment on the choice of research approach. Was a qualitative research approach suitable for the phenomenon being studied? In your opinion, would a more quantitative research approach have been more appropriate.

b. The data in the study were collected by observations and informal interviewing. Could the data have been collected in another way? Should they have been?

c. What type of sampling plan was used to sample observations in the study? Would an alternative sampling plan have been better? Why or why not?

d. The researcher recorded her observations, feelings, and interviews immediately after each 2-hour observation period. Comment on the appropriateness of this method. Can you identify any biases that could be present in this choice of method? Suggest alternative ways of recording the data.

e. How did the researcher handle the concept of saturation? Could you recommend any improvements?

f. What types of validation procedures did the researcher use? Can you suggest additional procedures that might have improved the study?

g. Comment on the thematic categories that emerged from the data. Do they seem to reflect accurately the data that were collected? Would you have developed different ones?

2. Below are several suggested research articles. Skim one of these articles and respond to relevant parts of Question D.1 in terms of an actual research study.
   - Grobe, S. J., Drew, J. A., & Fonteyn, M. E. (1991). A descriptive analysis of experienced nurses' clinical reasoning during a planning task. *Research in Nursing and Health, 14,* 305–314.
   - Mirr, M. P. (1991). Factors affecting decisions made by family members of patients with severe head injury. *Heart and Lung, 20,* 228–235.
   - Rather, M. L. (1992). "Nursing as a way of thinking"—Heideggerian hermeneutical analysis of the lived experience of the returning RN. *Research in Nursing and Health, 15,* 47–56.
   - Spitzer, A. (1992). Coping processes of school-age children with hemophilia. *Western Journal of Nursing Research, 14,* 157–168.

3. Lynch (1993)* conducted a study to investigate breastfeeding practices among teenaged mothers, who have been found in many studies to be less likely than older mothers to breastfeed. Using birth records from two large hospitals, Lynch contacted 250 young women between the ages of 15 and 19 who had given birth in the previous year and invited them to participate in a survey. Those who agreed to participate ($N = 185$) were interviewed by telephone (when possible), using a structured interview that asked about breastfeeding practices, attitudes toward motherhood, availability of social supports, and conflicting demands, such as school attendance or employment. Several psychologic scales (including measures of depression and self-esteem) were also administered. Teenagers without a telephone were interviewed in person in their own homes. All the teenagers interviewed at home were also interviewed in greater depth, using a topic guide that focused on such areas as feeling about breastfeeding, the decision-making process that led them to decide whether or not to breastfeed, barriers to breastfeeding, and intentions to breastfeed with any subsequent children. Lynch used the quantitative data to determine the characteristics associated with breastfeeding status and duration. The qualitative data were used to interpret and validate the quantitative findings.

   Review and critique this study. Suggest alternative data collection and analysis approaches. To assist you in your critique, here are some guiding questions.
   a. Which of the aims of integration, if any, were served by this study?
   b. What was the researcher's basic strategy for integration? How effective was this strategy in addressing the aims of integration?

---

*This example is fictitious.

    c. Suggest ways of altering the design of the study and the data collection approach to further promote integrative aims.

    d. Would the study have been stronger if it had involved the collection of quantitative data only? Qualitative data only? Why or why not?

4. Below are several suggested research articles of studies that used an integrated approach. Read one or more of these articles and respond to parts **a** to **d** of Question D.3 in terms of these actual research studies.

- Carrieri, V. K., Kieckhefer, G., Janson-Bjerklie, S., & Souza, J. (1991). The sensation of pulmonary dyspnea in school-age children. *Nursing Research, 40,* 81–85.

- Laffrey, S. C., & Pollock, S. E. (1990). An exploration of adult health behaviors. *Western Journal of Nursing Research, 12,* 434–446.

- Smith, C. E., Mayer, L. S., Parkhurst, C., Perkins, S. B., & Pingleton, S. K. (1991). Adaptation in families with a member requiring mechanical ventilation at home. *Heart and Lung, 20,* 349–356.

- Sohier, R. (1988). Multiple triangulation and contemporary nursing research. *Western Journal of Nursing Research, 10,* 732–742.

▌ E. SPECIAL PROJECTS

1. Get 10 or so people to write one or two paragraphs on their concerns about rising health care costs. Perform a thematic analysis of these paragraphs.

2. Develop two or three research questions that you think might lend themselves to a qualitative study.

3. Read one of the studies listed in the Suggested Readings of Chapter 11. Generate several hypotheses based on the reported findings.

4. Prepare three problem statements that would be amenable to multimethod research. For one of these research problems, write a two- to three-page description of how the data would be collected and how the use of both qualitative and quantitative data would strengthen the study.

Ethics, Critical Appraisal, and Utilization of Nursing Research

Part VI

|||||| Chapter 12
Ethics and Nursing Research

|| A. MATCHING EXERCISES

1. Match each of the descriptions in Set B with one of the procedures used to safeguard human subjects from Set A. Indicate the letter corresponding to the appropriate response next to each entry in Set B.

Set A

a. Freedom from harm or exploitation
b. Informed consent
c. Anonymity
d. Confidentiality

Set B   *Responses*

1. A questionnaire distributed by mail bears an identification number in one corner. Respondents are assured their responses will not be individually divulged.   _____
2. Hospitalized children included in a study, and their parents, are told the aims and procedures of the research. Parents are asked to sign an authorization.   _____
3. Respondents in a questionnaire study, in which the same respondents will be questioned twice, are asked to place their own four-digit identification number on the questionnaire and to memorize the number. Respondents are assured their answers will remain private.   _____
4. Women who recently had a mastectomy are studied in terms of psychological sequelae. In the interview, sensitive questions are carefully worded. After the interview, debriefing with the respondent determines the need for psychological support.   _____
5. Women interviewed in the above study (number 4) are told that the information they provide will not be individually divulged.   _____
6. Subjects who volunteered for an experimental treatment for AIDS are warned of potential side effects and are asked to sign a waiver.   _____

7. After determining that a new intervention resulted in discomfort to subjects, the researcher discontinued the study.   _____

8. Unmarked questionnaires are distributed to a class of nursing students. The instructions indicate that the responses will not be individually divulged.   _____

9. The researcher assures subjects that they will be interviewed as part of the study at a single point in time and adheres to this promise.   _____

10. A questionnaire distributed to a sample of nursing students includes a statement indicating that completion and submission of the questionnaire will be construed as voluntary participation in a study, as fully described in an accompanying letter.   _____

▌ B. COMPLETION EXERCISES

Write the words or phrases that correctly complete the sentences below.

1. Ethical _____ arise when the rights of subjects and the demands of science are put into direct conflict.

2. One of the first internationally recognized efforts to establish ethical standards was the _____.

3. The National Commission for the Protection of Human Subjects of Biomedical and Behavioral Research issued a well-known set of guidelines known as the _____.

4. The most straightforward ethical precept is the protection of subjects from _____.

5. Risks that are no greater than those ordinarily encountered in daily life are referred to as _____.

6. The right to _____ means that prospective subjects have the right to voluntarily decide whether or not to participate in a study, without risk of penalty.

7. The researcher adheres to the principle of _____ by fully describing to subjects the nature of the study and the likely risks and benefits of participation.

8. When the researcher cannot link research information to the person who provided it, the condition known as _____ has prevailed.

9. Special procedures are often required to safeguard the rights of _____ subjects.

10. Committees established in institutions to review proposed research procedures
    with respect to their adherence to ethical guidelines are often called IRBs, or
    _____.

‖ C. STUDY QUESTIONS

1. Define the following terms. Use the textbook to compare your definition with
   the definition in Chapter 12 or in the Glossary.

a. Code of ethics: _____

_____

_____.

b. Beneficence: _____

_____

_____.

c. Subject stipends: _____

_____

_____.

d. Debriefing: _____

_____

_____.

e. Risk/benefit ratio: _____

_____

_____.

f. Coercion: _____

_____

_____.

g. Covert data collection: _____

_____

_____.

h. Deception: _____

_____

_____.

i. Confidentiality: _____

_____

_____.

j. Informed consent: _____

_____

_____.

k. Vulnerable subjects: _____

_____

_____ .

2. Below are descriptions of several research studies. Suggest some ethical dilemmas that might emerge for each.

a. A study of coping behaviors among rape victims:

_____

_____

b. An unobtrusive observational study of fathers' behaviors in the delivery room:

_____

_____

c. An interview study of the antecedents of heroin addiction:

_____

_____

d. An investigation of the contraceptive decisions of adolescents (minors) using a family planning clinic:

_____

_____

e. An investigation of the verbal interactions among schizophrenic patients:

_____

_____

f. A study of the effects of a new drug on human subjects:

_____

_____

3. The following two studies involved the use of vulnerable subjects. Evaluate the ethical aspects of one or both of these studies, paying special attention to the manner in which the subjects' heightened vulnerability was handled.
   - Archbold, P. G., Stewart, B. J., Greenlick, M. R., & Harvath, T. (1990). Mutuality and preparedness as predictors of caregiver role strain. *Research in Nursing and Health, 13,* 375–383.
   - Nyamathi, A. M. (1991). Relationship of resources to emotional distress, somatic complaints, and high-risk behaviors in drug recovery and homeless minority women. *Research in Nursing and Health, 14,* 269–277.

4. In Chapter 12 of the textbook, two unethical studies were described (the study of syphilis among black men and the study in which live cancer cells were injected in elderly patients). Identify which ethical principles were transgressed in these studies.

5. A stipend of $5.00 was paid to the subjects completing a questionnaire on breastfeeding in the following study:

- Hill, P. D. (1991). Predictcors of breastfeeding duration among WIC and non-WIC mothers. *Public Health Nursing, 8,* 46–52.

Read the introductory sections of the report and comment on the appropriateness of the stipend.

6. Comment on the risk/benefit ratio and other ethical aspects of the following study, in which a mild form of deception was used:

- Forrester, D. A. (1990). AIDS-related risk factors, medical diagnosis, do-not-resuscitate orders and aggressiveness of nursing care. *Nursing Research, 39,* 350–354.

▌ D. APPLICATION EXERCISES

1. Kelley (1993)* investigated the behavior of nursing students in crisis or emergency situations. The investigator was interested in comparing the behaviors of students from baccalaureate versus diploma programs to determine the adequacy of the preparation given to students in handling emergencies. Fifty students from both types of programs volunteered to participate in the study. The investigator wanted to observe reactions to crises as they might occur naturally, so the participants were not told the exact nature of the study. Each student was instructed to take the vital signs of a "patient," purportedly to evaluate the students' skills. The "patient," who was described as another student but who in fact was a confederate of the investigator, simulated an epileptic seizure while the vital signs were being taken. A research assistant, who was unaware of the purpose of the study and who did not know the educational background of the subjects, observed the timeliness and appropriateness of the students' responses through a one-way mirror. Subjects were not required to divulge their identities. Immediately after participation, subjects were debriefed as to the true nature of the study and were paid a $10 stipend.

---

*This example is fictitious.

Consider the aspects of this study in regard to the issues discussed in this chapter. To assist in your review, you can answer the questions below, as well as the questions in Box 12-2 of the textbook.

  a. Were the subjects in this study at risk of physical or psychological harm? Were they at risk of exploitation?

  b. Did the subjects in the study derive any benefits from their participation? Did the nursing community or society at large benefit? How would you assess the risk/benefit ratio?

  c. Were the subjects' rights to self-determination violated? Was there any coercion involved? Was full disclosure made to subjects before participation? Was informed consent given to subjects and documented?

  d. Were subjects treated fairly? Was their right to privacy protected?

  e. What ethical dilemmas does this study present? How, if at all, can the dilemmas be resolved? To what extent *were* they resolved?

  f. What type of human subjects review would be appropriate for a study such as the one described?

2. Read one or more of the articles listed below. Respond to parts **a** to **f** of Question D.1 (as well as questions from Box 12-2 of the textbook) in terms of these actual research studies.

  ▪ Algase, D. L. (1992). Cognitive discriminants of wandering among nursing home residents. *Nursing Research, 41,* 78–81.

  ▪ Berger, M. C., Seversen, A., & Chvatal, R. (1991). Ethical issues in nursing. *Western Journal of Nursing Research, 13,* 514–521.

  ▪ Marchette, L., Main, R., Redick, E., Bagg, A., & Leatherland, J. (1991). Pain reduction interventions during neonatal circumcision. *Nursing Research, 40,* 241–244.

  ▪ Moody, L., McCormick, K., & Williams, A. R. (1991). Psychophysiologic correlates of quality of life in chronic bronchitis and emphysema. *Western Journal of Nursing Research, 13,* 336–352.

  ▪ Robichaud-Ekstrand, S. (1991). Shower versus sink bath: Evaluation of heart rate, blood pressure, and subjective response of the patient with myocardial infarction. *Heart and Lung, 20,* 375–381.

▌ E. SPECIAL PROJECTS

1. Prepare a brief summary of a hypothetical study in which the costs and benefits were both high. When the costs and benefits are essentially balanced, how should the researcher decide whether or not to proceed?

2. Skim the following research report, and draft an informed consent form for this study.

  ▪ Samselle, C. M., & DeLancey, J. O. L. (1992). The urine stream interruption test and pelvic muscle function. *Nursing Research, 41,* 73–77.

|||||| Chapter 13
Critiquing Research Reports

|| A. MATCHING EXERCISES

1. Match each of the questions in Set B with the research decision being evaluated, as listed in Set A. Indicate the letter(s) corresponding to your response next to each of the statements in Set B.

Set A

a. Evaluating the research design decisions
b. Evaluating the population and sampling plan
c. Evaluating the data collection procedures
d. Evaluating the analytic decisions

Set B	Responses
1. Were there a sufficient number of subjects?	_____
2. Was there evidence of adequate reliability and validity?	_____
3. Would a more limited specification have controlled some extraneous variables not covered by the research design?	_____
4. Would nonparametric tests have been more appropriate?	_____
5. Were respondents assured anonymity or confidentiality?	_____
6. Were threats to internal validity adequately controlled?	_____
7. Were the statistical tests appropriate, given the level of measurement of the variables?	_____
8. Were response set biases minimized?	_____
9. Was the comparison group equivalent to the experimental group?	_____
10. Should the data have been collected prospectively?	_____
11. Were triangulation procedures used as a method of validation?	_____
12. Were constant comparison procedures appropriately used to refine relevant categories?	_____
13. Did the researcher stay in the field long enough to gain an emic perspective?	_____
14. Were informants asked to comment on the emerging themes?	_____

▌ B. COMPLETION EXERCISES

1. The first step in the interpretation of research findings involves an analysis of the _____ of the results, based on various types of evidence.

2. Interpretation of results is easiest when the results are consistent with the researcher's _____.

3. An important research precept is that correlation does not prove _____.

4. Researchers should avoid the temptation of going beyond _____.

5. Statistical significance does not necessarily mean that research results are _____.

6. The research process involves numerous methodologic _____, each of which could affect the quality of the study.

7. A good critique should identify both _____ and _____ in a scientific study.

8. An evaluation of the relevance of a study to some aspect of the nursing profession involves critiquing the _____ dimension of a research study.

9. An evaluation of the researcher's plan to avoid self-selection biases involves critiquing the _____ dimension of a research study.

10. An evaluation of the way in which human subjects were treated involves critiquing the _____ dimension of a research study.

11. An evaluation of the sense the researcher tried to make of the results involves critiquing the _____ dimension of the research study.

12. An evaluation of the objectivity of the research report involves critiquing the _____ dimension of the research study.

▌ C. STUDY QUESTIONS

1. Define the following terms. Use the textbook to compare your definitions with the definitions in Chapter 13 or in the Glossary.

   a. Critique: _____

   _____

   _____

   b. Research decisions: _____

   _____

   _____

   c. Interpretation of results: _____

   _____

   _____

   d. Unhypothesized results: _____

   _____

   _____

2. Read the research report by Gretchen Randolph entitled "Therapeutic and physical touch: Physiological response to stressful stimuli," which appeared in the January 1984 issue of *Nursing Research* (volume 33, pages 33–36). None of the researcher's hypotheses were supported. Review and critique Randolph's interpretations of the findings and suggest some possible alternative explanations.

3. Below are several suggested research reports for studies in which the researcher obtained mixed results—that is, some hypotheses were supported and others were not. Review and critique the researcher's interpretation of the findings for one of these studies, and suggest possible alternatives.
   - Miller, K. M., & Perry, P. A. (1990). Relaxation technique and postoperative pain in patients undergoing cardiac surgery. *Heart and Lung, 19,* 136–146.
   - Naylor, M. D. (1990). Comprehensive discharge planning for hospitalized elderly: A pilot study. *Nursing Research, 39,* 156–161.
   - White, M. A., Williams, P. D., Alexander, D. J., Powell-Cope, G. M., & Conlon, M. (1990). Sleep onset latency and distress in hospitalized children. *Nursing Research, 39,* 134–139.

▌ D. APPLICATION EXERCISES

1. At the end of this Study Guide, in Part VII, are two actual research reports. Read one or both of these reports and prepare a three- to five-page critique summarizing the major strengths and weaknesses of the study.

▌ E. SPECIAL PROJECTS

1. Suppose that you were studying maternal behavior in mothers of normal and handicapped children. Fifty mothers from each group are observed interacting with their children (aged 7 to 10 years) in a laboratory setting for 30 minutes. Some data are presented below:

	Mothers with Normal Children	Mothers with Handicapped Children	t	p
Mean no. of times mother intiates conversations	10.2	12.8	2.3	<.05
Mean no. of minutes of silence	14.9	13.8	1.7	NS
Mean no. of times mother laughs or smiles	8.4	7.9	1.2	NS
Mean no. of direct maternal commands	8.7	6.1	3.8	<.05
Mean no. of encouraging/supportive comments	4.1	5.7	2.4	<.05

Write brief results and discussion sections for these data.

2. Rewrite Nelson's report (Chapter 13 of the text) using some of the suggestions from the critique in the textbook or from classroom discussions.

IIIIII Chapter 14
Utilization of Nursing Research

II A. MATCHING EXERCISES

1. Match each of the strategies from Set B with one of the roles indicated in Set A. Indicate the letters corresponding to your response next to each of the strategies in Set B.

Set A

a. Nurse researchers
b. Practicing nurses/nursing students
c. Nursing administrators

Set B   *Responses*

1. Become involved in a journal club   _____
2. Perform replications   _____
3. Offer resources for utilization projects   _____
4. Disseminate findings   _____
5. Specify clinical implications of findings   _____
6. Read research reports critically   _____
7. Foster intellectual curiosity in the work environment   _____
8. Provide a forum for communication between clinicians and
   researchers   _____
9. Expect evidence that a procedure is effective   _____
10. Attend nursing conferences and research sessions   _____

II B. COMPLETION EXERCISES

Write the words or phrases that correctly complete the sentences below.

1. _____ refers to the use of some aspect of a
   scientific investigation in an application unrelated to the original research.

2. There is considerable concern about the _____
   between knowledge production and knowledge utilization.

3. The most well-known nursing research utilization project, conducted in Michigan, is the _____ Project.

4. An early regional collaborative utilization project was the _____ _____ Project.

5. In order for research results to be believable, study findings must be _____ _____ in several different settings.

6. The three broad classes of criteria for research utilization are clinical relevance, scientific merit, and _____ .

7. The issue of _____ concerns whether it makes sense to implement an innovation in a new practice setting.

8. A cost/benefit ratio assessment should consider not only the net cost and gain of implementing an innovation but also _____ .

▮ C. STUDY QUESTIONS

1. Define the following terms. Use the textbook to compare your definition with the definition in Chapter 14 or in the Glossary.

a. Instrumental utilization: _____

_____

_____

b. Conceptual utilization: _____

_____

_____

c. Knowledge creep: _____

_____

_____

d. Decision accretion: _____

_____

_____

e. Awareness stage of adoption: _____

_____

_____

f. Persuasion stage of adoption: _____

_____

_____

g. Meta-analysis: _____

_____

_____

   h. Research proposals: _____

   _____

   _____

   i. Scientific merit: _____

   _____

   _____

   j. Cost/benefit ratio: _____

   _____

   _____

2. Prepare an example of a research question that could be posed to improve nursing care in the five phases of the nursing process.

   a. Assessment phase:

   _____

   _____

   b. Diagnosis phase:

   _____

   _____

   c. Planning phase:

   _____

   _____

   d. Intervention phase:

   _____

   _____

   e. Evaluation phase:

   _____

   _____

3. Think about a nursing procedure about which you have been instructed. What is the basis for this procedure? Determine whether the procedure is based on scientific evidence that the procedure is effective. If it is not based on scientific evidence, on what is it based, and why do you think scientific evidence was not used?

4. Identify the factors in your own setting that you think facilitate or inhibit research utilization (or, in an education setting, the factors that promote or inhibit a climate in which research utilization is valued).

5. Read Brett's (1987) article regarding the adoption of 14 nursing innovations ("Use of nursing practice research findings," *Nursing Research, 36,* 344–349), or read the more recent study based on the same 14 innovations by Coyle and Sokop (1990) ("Innovation adoption behavior among nurses," *Nursing Research, 39,* 176–180). For each of the 14 innovations, indicate whether you: are aware of the findings; are persuaded that the findings should be used; use the findings sometimes in a clinical situation; or use the findings always in a clinical situation.

1. _____
2. _____
3. _____
4. _____
5. _____
6. _____
7. _____
8. _____
9. _____
10. _____
11. _____
12. _____
13. _____
14. _____

6. With regard to the 14 innovations in Brett's study (see Question C.5 above), select an innovation or finding of which you (or most class members) were not aware. Go to the original source and read the research report. Perform a critique of the study, indicating in particular why you think there may have been barriers to having the innovation implemented in a local setting.

▌ D. APPLICATION EXERCISES

1. Below are several suggested research articles. Read one or more of these articles, paying special attention to the conclusion or implications section of the report. Evaluate the extent to which the researcher(s) facilitated the utilization of the study findings within clinical settings. If possible, suggest some clinical implications that the researchers did not discuss, or discuss the implications in terms of nursing education.

   - Fleury, J. D. (1991). Wellness motivation in cardiac rehabilitation. *Heart and Lung, 20,* 3–8.
   - Kruger, S. (1991). The patient educator role in nursing. *Applied Nursing Research, 4,* 19–23.
   - Lauver, D., & Rubin, M. (1991). Women's concerns about abnormal papanicolaou test results. *Journal of Obstetric, Gynecologic, and Neonatal Nursing, 20,* 154–159.
   - Maas, M. L., Buckwalter, K. C., & Kelley, L. S. (1991). Family members' perceptions of care of institutionalized patients with Alzheimer's disease. *Applied Nursing Research, 4,* 135–137.
   - Saudia, T. L., Kinney, M. R., Brown, K. C., & Young-Ward, L. (1991). Health locus of control and helpfulness of prayer. *Heart and Lung, 20,* 60–65.
   - Stone, K. S., Bell, S. D., & Preusser, B. A. (1991). The effect of repeated endotracheal suctioning on arterial blood pressure. *Applied Nursing Research, 4,* 152–158.

▌ E. SPECIAL PROJECTS

1. Select a study from the nursing research literature. Using the utilization criteria indicated in Boxes 14-1 and 14-2 of the text, assess the potential for utilizing the study results in a clinical practice setting. If the study meets the major criteria for utilization, develop a utilization plan.

Research Reports

Part VII

Gender Stereotyping and Nursing Care*

Deborah Dillon McDonald
and R. Gary Bridge†

The effect of gender stereotyping on nursing care was examined. Eight conditions were created in a posttest-only experiment by completely crossing patient gender (male/female) by memory load (low/ high) by patient health status (stable/unstable). One hundred sixty nurses read the same patient vignette. The vignette differed in patient gender, memory load, and patient health status. The nurses then estimated the minutes needed for specific nursing interventions with the patient. Nurses planned significantly more ambulation, analgesic administration, and emotional support time for the male patient, despite the presence of individuating information. More accurate, effective nursing care is possible when nurses are aware of the effect of gender stereotyping on nursing care.

Nurses strive to provide nursing care that optimizes their patients' health outcomes. In order to achieve this, nurses must accurately perceive their patients. The more accurately nurses perceive their patients, the more likely nurses are to use effective interventions to meet their patients' health needs. Attending to gender cues when gender is irrelevant to the situation is one source of perceptual inaccuracy. In this study gender stereotyping is approached from a cognitive perspective, and the effect of gender stereotyping on nursing care is examined.

Background

Integral to the perception of others is the need to make inferences about the other person. Bruner and Tagiuri (1954) describe Implicit Personality Theory (IPT), a

*This research was supported by the National Center for Nursing Research, NIH, Grant No. 5 F31 NR06168-02.

Reprinted here from *Research in Nursing and Health* (1991; 14:373–387), with permission.

†Deborah Dillon McDonald, PhD, RN, is an assistant professor in the School of Nursing, University of Connecticut. R. Gary Bridge, PhD, is an associate professor of psychology and education at Teachers College, Columbia University, New York.

"common-sense" theory of personality, as the process of making inferences about a person based on some external cue(s). Gender is an available and frequently used external cue in person perception (Ashmore & Del Boca, 1979).

Two assumptions about IPT make it an elegant way to examine gender stereotyping. First, the perceiver is often unaware that he or she is stereotyping because the influence is implicit (Cronbach, 1955). Second, gender stereotyping is a purely cognitive function, with no affective component (Miller, 1986). These two assumptions are absent in sociocultural theories of gender stereotyping. Both help distinguish gender stereotyping from sexual prejudice.

It is also important to distinguish functional gender stereotyping from dysfunctional gender stereotyping. Functional gender stereotyping occurs when the stereotype accurately reflects the current reality. Gender stereotyping under these circumstances simplifies information processing without decreasing the accuracy of the information. When the stereotype does not accurately reflect the current reality, inaccurate perceptions occur, and may lead to actions that are harmful to the perceived person.

Gender stereotyping of patients by nurses is crucial to examine, given the potential effect on patients' health outcomes. Ganong, Bzdek, and Manderino (1987) reviewed 38 studies of stereotyping by nurses and found only four studies that examined gender stereotyping. The four studies (Cowan, 1981; Kjervik, & Plata, 1978; Wallston, DeVellis, & Wallston, 1983; Worsley, 1980) were descriptive studies of attitudes. The studies were so diverse in methods and results that Ganong et al. (1987) were unable to draw any joint conclusions from them.

A review of gender stereotyping by health professionals supports the view that health professionals do gender stereotype. Fifteen out of 32 studies supported the proposition of gender stereotyping (Armitage, Schneiderman, & Bass, 1979; Aslin, 1977; Broverman, Broverman, Clarkson, Rosenkrantz, & Vogel, 1970; Cooperstock, 1971; Hamilton, Rothbart, & Dawes, 1986; Hohmann, 1989; Loring & Powell, 1988; Norwacki & Poe, 1973; O'Malley & Richarson, 1985; Phillips & Gilroy, 1985; Swenson & Ragucci, 1984; Vannicelli & Hamilton, 1984; Verbrugge & Steiner, 1984; Wallston et al., 1983; Worsley, 1980). Six studies did not support gender stereotyping by health professionals (Billingsley, 1977; Brems & Schlottmann, 1987; Glanz, Ganong, & Coleman, 1989; Kjervik & Palta, 1978; Marwit, 1981; Widiger & Settle, 1987). Kjervik and Palta's (1978) findings must be qualified with the fact that their sample consisted entirely of nurses with advanced degrees. It is not possible to generalize these findings to the general nursing population. The remaining 11 studies had method problems that prohibited interpretation of the results (Abramowitz et al., 1976; APA Task Force on Sex Bias, 1975; Colameco, Becker, & Simpson, 1983; Dreman, 1978; Gomes & Abramowitz, 1976; Kabacoff, Marwit, & Orlofsky, 1985; Marwit, 1981; Masling & Harris, 1969; McCranie, Horowitz, & Martin, 1978; Nalven, Hofman, & Bierbryer, 1969; Schwartz & Abramowitz, 1975; Smith, 1974).

Four method problems plague the gender stereotyping literature. First, the Sex Role Stereotyping Questionnaire (e.g., Broverman et al., 1970) has been used in many studies, but contains an imbalanced ratio of male to female valued items.

When this ratio was reversed, the direction of the sex bias also changed (Widiger & Settle, 1987). Second, many survey studies have a low survey response rate (e.g., APA Task Force on Sex Bias, 1975, 16% response rate). Third, many studies have selection and other internal validity threats from nonrandom assignment (e.g., Brems & Schlottmann, 1987), and use of nonrandom survey sampling (e.g., Swenson & Ragucci, 1984). Fourth, many investigators use thinly disguised manipulations that increase the likelihood of hypothesis guessing (e.g., Vannicelli & Hamilton, 1984). These pervasive method problems may explain why Smith's (1980) meta-analysis failed to support the thesis of gender stereotyping in mental health care.

It is important to take into account factors that may affect the potential to gender stereotype. Two factors, memory load and patient health status, may affect the likelihood of nurses to gender stereotype. When a patient's health status is unstable the patient is more likely to be perceived as distinctive. Consequently, the nurse is more likely to individuate the person and attend to information specific to that clinical problem. Locksley, Borgida, Brekke, and Hepburn (1980) found that as individuation increased, gender stereotyping decreased.

Memory load has the opposite effect. Memory load is the amount of information contained in short-term memory at a given point in time before being processed in long-term memory. Short-term memory capacity varies from person to person, but is generally limited to 7 ± 2 "chunks" of information (Carroll, 1986; Miller, 1956). This limitation forces people to simplify or categorize the information (Ashmore & Del Boca, 1979; Hamilton & Trolier, 1986; Taylor, Fiske, Etcoff, & Ruderman, 1978) into smaller, more manageable chunks. Categorizing people by gender was demonstrated experimentally by Taylor et al. (1978). Increased stereotyping as a result of increased memory load was demonstrated across three experiments by Rothbart, Fulerno, Jensen, and Birrell (1978). It follows that when nurses deal with a large amount of information (high memory load) they are more likely to stereotype.

In summary, the literature supports the hypothesis that health professionals gender stereotype. This literature is limited to findings such as gender differences in psychiatric diagnoses (Loring & Powell, 1988), psychotropic drug prescription (Hohmann, 1989), and workups for specific medical complaints (Armitage et al., 1979). There is no research on the specific effect of gender stereotyping on nursing care. An attempt to address this void was made in this study by testing the effect of gender stereotyping on five nursing interventions: patient ambulation and chair times, assessing comfort, analgesic administration, and emotional support.

❙❙ METHOD

This study was a posttest-only experiment with eight conditions created by a 2 (patient gender, male/female) by 2 (memory load, high/low) by 2 (patient health status, stable/unstable), completely crossed, between-subjects design.

Sample

One hundred sixty female medical–surgical registered nurses from the New England area were randomly assigned to the eight conditions. Their mean and median age was 33 and 29, respectively, with a standard deviation of 10.8, and a range of 21 to 67 years. By educational background 20.1% had associate degrees, 27% diplomas, 49.7% baccalaureate degrees, and 3.1% masters degrees. The percentage of full-time and part-time nurses was 81.2% and 18.8% respectively. The majority, 93.7%, were white. All the nurses worked in a teaching hospital at the time of the study.

Procedure

Nurses were tested individually or in groups following informed consent. The nurses were told that the study examined the way nurses think and organize their nursing care. Each nurse then received one of eight packets, corresponding to the eight experimental conditions. The packets were randomly ordered beforehand to avoid experimenter expectancy effects.

The experimental manipulation consisted of a written vignette about a 3-day postoperative colostomy patient. The vignette simulated a typical shift report for a medical–surgical patient. The vignette had been tested and judged an effective manipulation in a pilot study with 80 registered nurses.

The packets appeared identical, but differed in three ways: patient gender, memory load, and patient health status. The patient was named Mary B. in the feminine condition and Robert B. in the masculine condition. Nurses in the low memory load condition read only the colostomy patient vignette. Nurses in the high memory load condition read the same vignette, but as the fourth vignette among six others, each describing a different patient. Nurses in the high memory load condition were unaware of which patient they would be asked to respond to. Nurses in the unstable patient health status condition received the additional information that the patient's temperature had just spiked unexpectedly to 102°. Nurses read the vignette(s) with the expectation that they would plan nursing interventions for the patient during the next 8 hours. The vignette for the unstable feminine condition illustrates the information read by the nurses.

> *Mary B. is a 48-year-old with colon cancer. She had surgery 3 days ago creating a permanent colostomy. Today she says her pain is "8" (on a 1–10 scale with 1, no pain, and 10, unbearable pain). She has received Demerol 75 mg IM every 6 hours for the past 24 hours. Yesterday she was up to the chair 3 times for 30 minutes each, and walked in the hallway 3 times for 10 minutes each. Thirty minutes ago Mary's temperature spiked unexpectedly to 102°F.*

Nurses were instructed not to refer back to the vignette(s).

The nurses then responded to two manipulation checks. The memory load check asked how easy it was to recall all the information they had just read. The scale was a single 10-point bipolar scale with the anchors, *Very Easy* and *Very Difficult.* The manipulation check for patient health status asked the nurses to rate how important their nursing care would be for the patient. A 10-point bipolar scale was used with the anchors, *Very Important* and *Very Unimportant.*

Gender differentiated nursing interventions were measured in the following way. Nurses were instructed to estimate to the nearest minute the time they would plan for each of 16 relevant nursing actions. Five interventions were anticipated to show gender differences: patient ambulation, patient chair time, assessing comfort, analgesic administration, and emotional support. The remaining 11 interventions served as fillers to increase task realism and distract participants from the true purpose. These fillers consisted of generic physiologic responses and learning needs, and were not likely to be gender differentiated. The fillers consisted of assessing lungs, bowel sounds, skin, nutritional intake, signs of infection, colostomy and colostomy output, degree of abdominal distension, and teaching colostomy care, home care needs, and incisional splinting. Nurses completed a page of demographic information at the end of the experiment. They were then informed that the experiment was over and debriefed.

Analysis

Five full factorial analyses of variance (ANOVA) tested for gender differentiated nursing care, one for each of the five interventions. For example, the time nurses planned to ambulate the patient was entered as the dependent measure in a 2 (gender) × 2 (memory load) × 2 (patient status) ANOVA. Random assignment to the eight conditions was examined by separate ANOVA's for each of the demographic variables measured.

‖ RESULTS

No demographic differences between nurses in the eight conditions were found for age, marital status, ethnicity, educational background, or work experience. The manipulation checks yielded mixed results. The memory load manipulation was effective. Nurses in the high memory load condition had more difficulty recalling the patient information, $t(157) = 5.97$, $p < .001$, than nurses in the low memory load condition. The patient health status manipulation showed no differences between groups.

Gender differentiated nursing care occurred in three of the five anticipated nursing interventions: ambulation, analgesic administration, and emotional support. Nurses planned significantly more ambulation time, analgesic administration time, and emotional support time for the male. There were no significant two-way or three-way interaction effects between patient gender, memory load, or patient health status. Table 1 contains the means, standard deviations, and significance test results of the gender main effects for the five dependent variables. In contrast, a

Table 1. Time Planned for Nursing Interventions

	Nursing Care	Female	Male	F	df	p
Ambulate						
	M	14.7	18.3	4.84	1,151	.029
	SD	9.25	11.52			
	n	(79)	(80)			
Medicate						
	M	7.2	8.8	4.01	1,146	.047
	SD	3.94	5.75			
	n	(77)	(77)			
Support						
	M	18.4	25.4	5.14	1,144	.025
	SD	12.48	22.66			
	n	(77)	(76)			
Chair						
	M	43.4	49.0	1.40	1,148	.239
	SD	31.51	27.93			
	n	(77)	(79)			
Comfort						
	M	8.0	5.7	3.27	1,146	.073
	SD	9.96	4.85			
	n	(78)	(76)			

separate group of ANOVAs for the 11 fillers did not support any significant gender main effects.

▌ DISCUSSION

Nurses planned different care for a male and female patient in three of five anticipated nursing interventions despite the presence of relevant patient information. For example, even when informed that the patient had ambulated three times for 10 minutes each time during the previous 24 hr, nurses planned to ambulate the male patient 35% more than the female patient. This conflicts with Locksley, Borgida, Brekke, and Hepburn's (1980) finding that individuating information decreases stereotyping. These differences cannot be attributed to actual gender differences. Extraneous factors such as this were controlled by the study's experimental design. Low memory load and unstable patient health status also failed to deter the effect of gender stereotyping. This is suggested by the absence of interaction effects. The present study indicates the strength that gender stereotypes exert on nursing care.

Two of the five predicted interventions, patient chair time and assessing comfort, did not support gender stereotyping by nurses. Sitting in the chair generally requires less physical stamina than ambulating. This difference may explain why gender differences occurred with ambulation, but not chair times. Assessing comfort may be more a function of the nurse than the patient. Nurses may routinely assess pain responses when they are with the patient without regard to factors such as gender.

The impact on patient health outcomes from this gender differentiated care is important to consider. The three significant interventions—patient ambulation, analgesic administration, and emotional support—appear to favor the male patient. The effects of prolonged inactivity are known to decrease cardiovascular performance and diaphragmatic movement, and increase thromboembolic phenomena, decubitus ulcers, muscle weakness, and constipation (Halar & Bell, 1988). Appropriately administered analgesics promote comfort, decrease anxiety (McCaffery & Beebe, 1989), and allow mobility without severe additional pain. Emotional support often increases coping ability (Gottlieb, 1985). It is vital that women share equitably in the benefits of these nursing interventions.

While the internal validity of this experiment is relatively strong, the external validity is not. It is possible that the paper and pencil manipulation failed to elicit the effect of an actual social interaction. The manipulation was devoid of the usual verbal and nonverbal cues that occur during most nurse and patient interactions. These cues may be crucial in preventing gender stereotyping. If this is true, the external validity of these findings is greatly diminished. It is equally as important to point out that the manipulation also was devoid of the demand effects (Rosenthal, 1966; Snyder, 1984) that nurses may exhibit towards patients. The demand effect would encourage the patient to behave in a gender-stereotypic way. The exclusive testing of practicing nurses adds to the external validity of this study.

Results from this study indicate the need for research in seven areas. First, this study demonstrates that under experimental conditions, nurses planned different care for a male and female patient. The external validity of these results remains to be determined. This could be accomplished by a study in which medical records were reviewed or through the observation of nurses giving direct patient care. Second, other populations should be tested. Female medical–surgical registered nurses from New England were tested in this study. The results are generalizable only to this population. Nurses from other specialty areas, cultures, and geographic locations, as well as other health professionals and members of both genders should be tested. Third, a study in which the underlying reasons for gender differentiated care are addressed may help clarify some implicit misconceptions. Fourth, nursing care of patients with other health problems such as myocardial infarctions or chronic obstructive pulmonary disease should be examined. Fifth, other aspects of nursing care need to be tested. For example, does gender stereotyping affect the nurses' ability to develop a collaborative relationship with the patient? Sixth, educational efforts that decrease gender stereotyping and increase an androgynous perspective should be evaluated. Seventh, other stereotypes such as stereotypes of older adults and members of minority groups need to be tested.

Attending to gender cues when gender is irrelevant to the clinical situation is one source of perceptual inaccuracy for nurses. This study indicates that under experimental conditions, medical–surgical registered nurses do attend to irrelevant gender cues and plan gender differentiated nursing care. Identifying conditions in which gender stereotyping is likely to occur makes more accurate, effective nursing care possible.

REFERENCES

Abramowitz, S., Roback, H., Schwartz, J., Yasuma, A., Abramowitz, C., & Gomes, B. (1976). Sex bias in psychotherapy: A failure to confirm. *American Journal of Psychiatry, 133,* 706–709.

APA Task Force on Sex Bias. (1975). Report of the task force on sex bias and sex-role stereotyping in psychotherapeutic practice. *American Psychologist, 30,* 1169–1175.

Armitage, K., Schneiderman, L., & Bass, R. (1979). Response of physicians to medical complaints of men and women. *Journal of the American Medical Association, 241,* 2186–2187.

Ashmore, R., & Del Boca, F. (1979). Sex stereotypes and implicit personality theory: Toward a cognitive social psychological conceptualization. *Sex Roles, 5,* 219–248.

Aslin, A. (1977). Feminist and mental health center psychotherapists' expectations of mental health for women. *Sex Roles, 3,* 537–544.

Billingsley, D. (1977). Sex bias in psychotherapy: An examination of the effect of client sex, client pathology, and therapist sex on treatment planning. *Journal of Consulting and Clinical Psychology, 45,* 250–256.

Brems, C., & Schlottmann, R. (1987). Gender-bound definitions of mental health. *The Journal of Psychology, 122,* 5–14.

Broverman, I., Broverman, D., Clarkson, F., Rosenkrantz, P., & Vogel, S. (1970). Sex stereotypes and clinical judgments of mental health. *Journal of Consulting and Clinical Psychology, 34,* 1–7.

Bruner, J., & Tagiuri, R. (1954). The perception of people. In G. Lindzey (Ed.), *Handbook of social psychology* (pp. 634–654). Reading, MA: Addison-Wesley.

Carroll, D. (1986). *Psychology of language.* Pacific Grove, CA: Brooks/Cole.

Colameco, S., Becker, L., & Simpson, M. (1983). Sex bias in the assessment of patient complaints. *The Journal of Family Practice, 16,* 1117–1121.

Cooperstock, R. (1971). Sex differences in the use of mood-modifying drugs: An explanatory model. *Journal of Health and Social Behavior, 12,* 238–244.

Cowan, C. (1981). Sexism by nurses. *The Lamp, 38,* 5–12.

Cronbach, L. (1955). Processes affecting scores on "understanding of others" and "assumed similarity." *Psychological Bulletin, 52,* 177–193.

Dreman, S. (1978). Sex-role stereotyping in mental health standards in Israel. *Journal of Clinical Psychology, 34,* 961–966.

Ganong, L., Bzdek, V., & Manderino, M. (1987). Stereotyping by nurses and nursing students: A critical review of research. *Research in Nursing & Health, 10,* 49–70.

Glanz, D., Ganong, L., & Coleman, M. (1989). Client gender, diagnosis and family structure. *Western Journal of Nursing Research, 11,* 726–735.

Gomes, B., & Abramowitz, S. (1976). Sex-related patient and therapist effects on clinical judgment. *Sex Roles, 2,* 1–13.

Gottlieb, B. (1985). Social networks and social support: An overview of research, practice and policy implications. *Health Education Quarterly, 12,* 5–22.

Halar, E., & Bell, K. (1988). Contracture and other deleterious effects of immobility. In J. DeLisa (Ed.), *Rehabilitation medicine principles and practice.* Philadelphia: J.B. Lippincott.

Hamilton, D., & Trolier, T. (1986). Stereotypes and stereotyping: An overview of the cognitive approach. In J. F. Dovido & S. L. Gaertner (Eds.), *Prejudice, discrimination and racism* (pp. 127–163). New York: Academic Press.

Hamilton, S., Rothbart, M., & Dawes, R. (1986). Sex bias, diagnosis, and DSM-III. *Sex Roles, 15,* 269–274.

Hohmann, A. (1989). Gender bias in psychotropic drug prescribing in primary care. *Medical Care, 27,* 478–490.

Kabacoff, R., Marwit, S., & Orlofsky, J. (1985). Correlates of sex role stereotyping among mental health professionals. *Professional Psychology: Research and Practice, 16,* 98–105.

Kjervik, D., & Palta, M. (1978). Sex-role stereotyping in assessment of mental health. *Nursing Research, 16,* 98–105.

Locksley, A., Borgida, E., Brekke, N., & Hepburn, C. (1980). Sex stereotypes and social judgment. *Journal of Personality and Social Psychology, 39,* 821–831.

Loring, M., & Powell, B. (1988). Gender, race, and DSM-III: A study of the objectivity of psychiatric diagnostic behavior. *Journal of Health and Social Behavior, 29,* 1–22.

Marwit, S. (1981). Assessment of sex-role stereotyping among male and female psychologist practitioners. *Journal of Personality Assessment, 45,* 593–599.

Masling, J., & Harris, S. (1969). Sexual aspects of TAT administration. *Journal of Consulting and Clinical Psychology, 33,* 166–169.

McCaffery, M., & Beebe, A. (1989). *Pain clinical manual for nursing practice.* Philadelphia: C. V. Mosby.

McCranie, E., Horowitz, A., & Martin, R. (1978). Alleged sex-role stereotyping in the assessment of women's physical complaints: A study of general practitioners. *Social Science and Medicine, 12,* 111–116.

Miller, C. (1986). Categorization and stereotyping about men and women. *Personality and Social Psychology Bulletin, 12,* 502–512.

Miller, G. (1956). The magical number seven, plus or minus two: Some limits on capacity for processing information. *Psychological Review, 63,* 81–97.

Nalven, F., Hofman, L., & Bierbryer, B. (1969). Effects of subjects' age, sex, race, and socioeconomic status on psychologists' estimates of "true IQ" from WISC scores. *Journal of Clinical Psychology, 25,* 271–274.

Norwacki, C., & Poe, C. (1973). The concept of mental health as related to sex of person perceived. *Journal of Counseling and Clinical Psychology, 40,* 160.

O'Malley, K., & Richardson, S. (1985). Sex bias in counseling: Have things changed? *Journal of Counseling and Development, 63,* 294–299.

Phillips, R., & Gilroy, F. (1985). Sex role stereotypes and clinical judgments of mental health: The Brovermans' findings reexamined. *Sex Roles, 12,* 179–193.

Rosenthal, R. (1966). *Experimenter effects in behavioral research.* New York: Appleton-Century-Crofts.

Rothbart, M., Fulero, S., Jensen, C., Howard, J., & Birrell, P. (1978). From individual to group impressions: Availability heuristic in stereotype formation. *Journal of Experimental and Social Psychology, 14,* 237–255.

Schwartz, J., & Abramowitz, S. (1975). Value-related effects on psychiatric judgment. *Archives of General Psychiatry, 32,* 1525–1529.

Smith, M. (1974). Influence of client sex and ethnic group on counselor judgments. *Journal of Counseling Psychology, 21,* 516–521.

Smith, M. (1980). Sex bias in counseling and psychotherapy. *Psychological Bulletin, 87,* 392–407.

Snyder, M. (1984). When beliefs create reality. In L. Berkowitz (Ed.), *Advances in experimental social psychology* (pp. 247–303). New York: Academic Press.

Swenson, E., & Ragucci, R. (1984). Effects of sex-role stereotypes and androgynous alternatives of mental health judgments of psychotherapists. *Psychological Reports, 54,* 475–481.

Taylor, S., Fiske, S., Etcoff, N., & Ruderman, A. (1978). Categorical and contextual bases of person memory and stereotyping. *Journal of Personality and Social Psychology, 36,* 778–793.

Vannicelli, M., & Hamilton, G. (1984). Sex-role values and bias in alcohol treatment personnel. *Cultural and Sociological Aspects of Alcoholism and Substance Abuse, 4,* 57–68.

Verbugge, L., & Steiner, R. (1984). Another look at physicians' treatment of men and women with common complaints. *Sex Roles, 11,* 1091–1109.

Wallston, B., DeVillis, B., & Wallston, K. (1983). Licensed practical nurses' sex role stereotypes. *Psychology of Women Quarterly, 7,* 199–208.

Widiger, T., & Settle, S. (1987). Broverman et al. revisited: An artifactual sex bias. *Journal of Personality and Social Psychology, 53,* 463–469.

Worsley, A. (1980). Exploration of student nurses' stereotypes of patients. *International Journal of Nursing Studies, 17,* 163–174.

AIDS Family Caregiving: Transitions Through Uncertainty*

Marie Annette Brown
and Gail M. Powell-Cope†

The purpose of this study was to describe the experience of AIDS family caregiving. Grounded theory provided the methodological basis for qualitative data generation and analysis. Extensive interviews were conducted with 53 individuals (lovers, spouses, parents of either adults or children with AIDS, siblings, and friends) who were taking care of a person with AIDS at home. Relevant features of the social context of AIDS family caregiving were explored. Findings revealed the basic social psychological problem of Uncertainty, a core category of Transitions Through Uncertainty, and five subcategories: Managing and Being Managed by the Illness; Living With Loss and Dying; Renegotiating the Relationship; Going Public; and Containing the Spread

*Accepted for publication April 8, 1991. Earlier versions of this paper were presented at the 1989 meeting of the Western Institute for Nursing and the 1989 Council of Nurse Researchers meeting. This study was funded in part by a Biomedical Research Support Grant from the University of Washington School of Nursing and the Psi Chapter of Sigma Theta Tau. Although there is a designated first and second author, this article is a result of a collaborative effort between the authors. Both authors contributed equally to the final product. We gratefully acknowledge the generous contribution of time from our study participants. We sincerely appreciate the substantive and methodological assistance provided by Kristen Swanson, PhD, RN, Phil Bereano, PhD, Kimberly Moody, PhC, RN, and Linda Meldman, PhC, RN.

Reprinted here from *Nursing Research* (1991;40[6]:338–345), with permission.

†Marie Annette Brown, PhD, RN, is an associate professor in the School of Nursing, University of Washington, Seattle, WA.

Gail M. Powell-Cope, PhC, RN, is a doctoral candiate in nursing science at the school of Nursing, University of Washington, Seattle, WA.

of HIV. Stages and strategies of each subcategory detailed individuals' responses to the challenges of AIDS family caregiving and elaborated the day-to-day experiences. Uncertainty as a critical challenge for individuals and families facing life-threatening illness is discussesd in light of recent research.

The physical and emotional devastation of HIV infection and AIDS produces extraordinary challenges to the health care system. Families and significant others assume heavy responsibilities for care of these individuals and provide the cornerstone of society's response to the AIDS epidemic (Haque, 1989; Wolcott et al., 1986). For example, Raveis and Siegel (1990) found that informal or familial caregivers provided approximately two-thirds of the total assistance required for instrumental activities, transportation, administrative activities, and home medical care for persons with AIDS (PWAs) even though the sample was relatively healthy. Hepburn (1990) emphasized that if family caregivers of PWAs "play a comparable role to informal caregivers of the elderly, they will have significant impact on the overall care and well-being of AIDS patients" (p. 41).

‖ LITERATURE REVIEW

The literature suggests that there are risks to assuming the family caregiver role of an elderly or ill person including physical morbidity (Snyder & Keefe, 1985; Baumgarten, 1989); depression, mental exhaustion, and burnout (Chenoweth & Spencer, 1986; Ekberg, Griffith, & Foxall, 1986; Livingston, 1985); burden, strain (Montgomery, Gonyea, & Hooyman, 1985; Zarit, Todd, & Zarit, 1986); anger, depression, fatigue (Rabins, Mace, & Lucas, 1982; Rabins, Fitting, Eastham, & Fettig, 1990); and uncertainty (Stetz, 1989). Furthermore, parent caregivers of chronically ill children experience changes in the marital relationship, financial constraints, and role alterations (Thomas, 1987). These parent caregivers often become socially isolated as they focus on the ill child, become less available for reciprocal exchange with others, and experience the withdrawal of friends and other family members (Thomas, 1987). It is particularly common that middle-aged caregivers are unable to fulfill their work and family roles adequately (Miller & Montgomery, 1990). In a recent study of informal caregivers of PWAs, alterations in work role performance and economic burden were common, even though the sample consisted of relatively healthy PWAs with few functional disabilities (Raveis & Siegel, 1990). Over one-third of the caregivers had made financial changes in their lives and passed up financial opportunities, and 13% reported somewhat serious financial problems. Most (72%) of those employed reported that their ability to concentrate at work was affected by the patient's illness. A substantial minority (39%) reported arriving at work late or leaving early because the PWA was ill, had to be escorted to a medical appointment, or needed assistance with errands. Twenty-eight percent admitted that in recent months they had to take sick leave, vacation, or personal days because of the PWA's illness (Raveis & Siegel, 1990).

While there may be challenges common for all caregivers, each subgroup of caregivers face unique psychosocial stressors, often related to the characteristics of the care recipient. Issues of communicability, stigma, and multiple and premature losses are common in AIDS family caregiving. The issue of communicability of this "deadly disease" can stimulate fears of contagion and death in loved ones, friends, and coworkers of both the patient and the family caregiver (Ostrow & Gayle, 1986). Coping with AIDS phobia, the stigma associated with homosexuality, bisexuality, or IV drug use, as well as the tremendous demands of caregiving, may become overwhelming for family members (Moffatt, 1986). Schoen (1986) highlighted the additional strain faced by younger caregivers, particularly spouses and lovers, who deal with such a catastrophic, life-threatening illness before reaching half of their life expectancy, and who have not acquired the maturity and perspective that often accompany middle and older age. Caregivers who are HIV positive witness deterioration and death that could forecast their own fate (Shilts, 1987; Edwards, 1988). Lastly, a large proportion of AIDS family caregivers are men, who in American culture usually receive less preparation than women for nurturing roles.

Virtually no information exists about AIDS family caregiving, and much of the general family caregiving research focuses only on caregiving tasks and related effects on the caregiver (Bowers, 1987). The grounded theory method is a particularly important research strategy to address these gaps and serves to "clarify, develop, or redirect research in a content area about which much is already known" (Bowers, 1987, p. 31). Therefore, the purpose of this grounded theory study was to explore and describe the experience of family members who were caring for PWAs at home. The term *family caregiver* employed in this study includes family of origin and family of choice.

▊ METHOD

Sample

Participants were recruited from a variety of AIDS community sources, including clinics, support groups, a caregiver course, volunteer organizations, and a community newspaper. The sample consisted of 53 family caregivers of people with symptomatic HIV infection or AIDS. Approximately one-third (32%) were partners or lovers in gay relationships, 6% were partners or spouses in heterosexual relationships, 43% were friends (9% were former lovers), 13% were parents, 4% were siblings, and 4% were other family of origin. The parents included those of both adult and minor children with HIV/AIDS. Seventy-seven percent lived in the same household with the PWA and 60% of the households also included other individuals such as the caregiver's partner, child, or housemate. Approximately two-thirds (64%) of the family caregivers were male and 36% were female. Approximately two-thirds (68%) were gay or bisexual and 32% were heterosexual. The sample ranged from 22 to 65 years old ($M = 36$). Fifty-seven percent had less than a college degree and 92% were white. Fifty percent of the caregivers were employed full-time and 19% part-time outside the home. Family incomes (which supported an average of 1.9 persons) were low, with 18% reporting under $10,000, 41% between $10–20,000, 16% $20–30,000, 16% $30–40,000, and 9% over $40,000. In almost half (47%) of the families, the PWA had been diagnosed within the past 12 months. Eighty-four percent of the caregivers knew the PWA prior to the diagnosis of AIDS. The sample contained few ethnic minorities and a large number of caregivers of gay PWAs, thus reflecting the demographics of AIDS in the geographical area where the study was conducted (DSHS & Seattle-King County Health Department, 1991). However, compared to family caregivers of people with other health problems, this sample was younger with a greater proportion of men, fewer spouses, and fewer members from families of origin.

Procedure

After consent was obtained, participants were asked: "What has it been like for you living with and taking care of someone with AIDS?" Relevant probes were used to gain further insight into issues raised. In addition, an interview guide was used to insure consistency of topics across interviews. Interviews were conducted in either one or two sessions, lasted a mean of 4.5 hours, and yielded over 200 hours of interview data. Confidentiality was maintained.

While a triangulation of methods was used to address the study purpose, this paper will include only findings from qualitative analyses. Grounded theory (Glaser & Strauss, 1967; Strauss, 1987) provided the methodological basis for qualitative data generation and analysis. This approach is derived from symbolic interactionism, which focuses on human social and psychological processes as they are grounded in social interaction. The basic tenet of symbolic interactionism is that people construct meanings about phenomenon based on interpretations of interactions they have with one another and with themselves (Blumer, 1969). Therefore, family caregiving is viewed as a socially interactive process that supports the ill person, in this case, the person with HIV infection.

Interviews were tape-recorded and transcribed verbatim. Constant comparative analysis was used as an ongoing technique that included deriving first level codes, or in vivo codes, comparing codes to one another, deriving conceptual categories, and relating categories to codes and to other categories. Coding strategies included open coding (unrestricted selection of codes from the search for words or phrases that capture the meaning in the transcripts), axial coding (comparison between codes), and selective coding (utilization of frequently occurring codes to create core categories). Theoretical sampling was accomplished by selecting respondents based on the need to collect more data to examine categories and their relationships, and to ensure representativeness in the category. Theoretical saturation determined the discontinuation of new data collection. Theoretical saturation occurred when information became redundant and a core category was created and linked to subcategories.

Validity and reliability of the data were addressed systematically using the criteria outlined by Sandelowski (1986) and Lincoln and Guba (1985): (a) truth value, (b) applicability, (c) consistency, and (d) neutrality. Member checks, debriefing by peers, triangulation, prolonged engagement with the data, persistent observation, and reflective journals were techniques used to ensure validity and reliability. During the final phases of analysis, focus groups of study alumni, family caregivers who did not participate in the study, and professionals and community volunteers working in the area of AIDS family caregiving were asked to review and to critique the validity of the substantive theory of AIDS family caregiving. Modifications of the theoretical presentation were made based on feedback from these experts as well as from consensus between the researchers. The categories developed during this study were also validated using literature in the popular press. Examination of Monette's (1988) detailed account of caring for his partner with AIDS revealed evidence of the basic social psychological problem, core category, subcategories, and stages and strategies.

Context and Assumptions

Grounded theory methodology suggests that it is crucial to examine the broader social context of the phenomenon under study. The data from this study represent caregiving that occurred between 1985 and 1988. Caregiving during those years of the AIDS epidemic was inextricably linked to several salient issues: a silent government, a vocal gay community, an unresponsive bureaucracy, inexperienced health care providers, and a frightened, uninformed, and homophobic populace.

Specific aspects of the cultural context can be related to the five subcategories describing caregivers' responses to the challenge of AIDS. For example, complicating the caregivers' attempt to manage the illness was a society that undervalued care provided in the home and traditionally expected women to fulfill that role without compensation or reward. Living with loss and dying was made more difficult by the high value placed on youth and appearance. Pervasive divorce and domestic violence as well as widespread intolerance of nontraditional family compositions undermined the ability to maintain relationships. Because of the societal stigma associated with AIDS and fear of exposure to prejudice, persons with AIDS and caregivers were not encouraged to "go public" with their disease, but instead had to hide the truth.

Moreover, the attempt to contain the spread of HIV was hindered by contradictory messages. On one hand, popular images promoted by the media and embraced by society suggested that romantic sex should ideally be spontaneous and unprotected. While on the other hand, the medical community advised condom use to prevent the transmission of AIDS. Yet despite the information provided by the medical community, their efforts to convince the general public to practice "safe" sex were not adequate.

‖ RESULTS

The substantive theory of AIDS family caregiving developed during this study is outlined in Figure 1. *Uncertainty* was identified as the basic social psychological problem and *Transitions Through Uncertainty* the core category of AIDS family caregiving. In addition to the pervasive sense of uncertainty that characterized the AIDS caregiving transition, the day-to-day experience of uncertainty was best understood in the context of the five caregiving subcategories (Figure 1). These subcategories provide a structure for detailing the multiple aspects of uncertainty. The subcategories also highlighted areas of caregivers' lives that were most significant and problematic. Stages and strategies of each subcategory detail caregivers' action-oriented responses to the uncertainties and specific challenges characteristic of each subcategory.

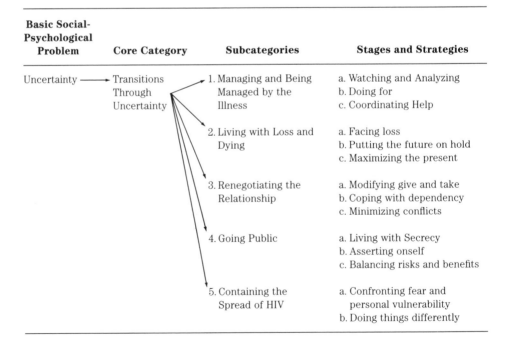

Basic Social-Psychological Problem	Core Category	Subcategories	Stages and Strategies
Uncertainty ⟶	Transitions Through Uncertainty	1. Managing and Being Managed by the Illness	a. Watching and Analyzing b. Doing for c. Coordinating Help
		2. Living with Loss and Dying	a. Facing loss b. Putting the future on hold c. Maximizing the present
		3. Renegotiating the Relationship	a. Modifying give and take b. Coping with dependency c. Minimizing conflicts
		4. Going Public	a. Living with Secrecy b. Asserting onself c. Balancing risks and benefits
		5. Containing the Spread of HIV	a. Confronting fear and personal vulnerability b. Doing things differently

Figure 1. Substantive Theory of AIDS Family Caregiving

Uncertainty[1]

Uncertainty was identified as the basic social psychological problem in the AIDS caregiving transition. Uncertainty, as conceptualized in this study, is defined as the caregiver's inability to predict future events and outcomes and the lack of confidence in making day-to-day decisions about the ill person's care. Uncertainty exerted a profound influence on caregivers' lives and pervaded the entire caregiving experience; it never completely disappeared, but varied in intensity, timing, and content. Even though caregivers reported increasing confidence in their caregiving abilities and increasing ability to predict outcomes over time, uncertainty about some issue always remained. Even after one year of caregiving, one lover expressed some self-doubts:

> *So I don't necessarily feel 100% about everything I'm doing, but I have to do it ... I'm not 100% positive, 100% sure, 100% that it's the right thing to do for Mike ... It becomes very obscure, blurry, as to whether I'm doing anything right.*

Feelings of uncertainty in AIDS family caregiving arose from the perpetual and unpredictable changes accompanying AIDS. The PWA's health or functional ability and the caregivers' emotional responses were often in a constant state of flux. One caregiver emphasized the difficulties in trying to keep abreast of these constant changes:

> *It constantly changes. I want to emphasize that. You can't learn what the boundary is, because the boundary of today is not gonna be the boundary of tomorrow. What you've got to learn is how to have an antenna.*

Often, study participants spontaneously offered the roller coaster metaphor to describe the constant changes inherent in AIDS caregiving. A roller coaster, with many ups and downs, reflected the relentlessness and the lack of control in AIDS family caregiving. For the most part, caregivers were unable to seek respite from the constant drama of AIDS, and to create a more stable period in the lives. Two different caregivers expressed their feelings about the roller coaster as follows:

> *The roller coaster describes the situation in lots of different ways. What's happening to the person's health? What's happening to your feelings? What's happened here today? It's this incredible uncertainty.*

> *Well, it got to be like an emotional roller coaster, one of these up and down and up and down ... So it's almost as*

---

[1]Although our analysis was conducted without knowledge of Mishel's reconceptualization of the uncertainty in illness theory (1990), the studies contain parallel findings that support an expanded perspective on the acceptance of uncertainty.

> *though you want to tell yourself, well, his condition is stabi-*
> *lized. This stuff doesn't stabilize very long...*

Uncertainty was problematic for caregivers because of a cultural context that emphasizes the need to understand, predict, and/or control events. Caregivers struggled as they faced the contradiction between their expectations about prediction and control and the reality of their personal experiences which were imbued with constant uncertainty. Initially, caregivers expected health care providers to be able to provide them with incontestable information about AIDS and the PWA's course of illness. Caregivers often were frustrated when they turned to health care providers for definitive answers and found that the professionals were themselves equally uncertain. One caregiver expressed his frustration with the inability of the physicians to explain his partner's new and foreboding neurological symptoms:

> *He's got a malfunction in his brain and no one knows*
> *what's going on. The neurosurgeons, and neurologists and*
> *doctors at the AIDS clinic ... No one knows what's happening,*
> *but it's getting worse.*

While some caregivers learned to accept uncertainty over time, others had a stronger need to establish some degree of certainty in their lives. Some caregivers did not want to accept the uncertainty of AIDS caregiving and tried to force certainty where it did not exist. After numerous attempts to exercise control in the face of constant change, many caregivers discovered the fallacy of this imperative and began to accept uncertainty. One caregiver poignantly described his paradoxical reflections about the uncertainty of his lover's mortality:

> *I like to know what's going to happen in a clear-cut path*
> *in a pattern that I can control ... So my certainty was that I*
> *finally decided Mike was going to die. Finally I realized what*
> *right do I have to decide the fate of someone else's life? He*
> *may not die. I was doing it for my own protection, my own*
> *sanity ... So I opened up that wound, or whatever you call*
> *that, and let uncertainty back into my life.*

Transitions

A transition is a period of major change in life circumstances accompanied by uncertainty, questioning one's basic assumptions, and reexamining plans for living in the world (Parkes, 1971) which results in the reordering of life activities and a transformed self-identity. As a result of prolonged engagement with the data and with the literature, we identified caregiving as a transition to be a critical feature of AIDS family caregiving. Study participants consistently described AIDS caregiving as a significant phase of life as portrayed in the definition above. Many emphasized caregiving as a process that occurred over time or a series of changes. This lover struggled with the effects of dramatic changes in the PWA's health over a short period of time:

> *You should have talked to me three months ago when he was in the hospital with pneumonia. Life was completely different then: I was a basket case, whirling from the news from AIDS and afraid of death at any moment. Now he's back to work and we seem to be pretending that we are living a normal life.*

Others viewed caregiving as a journey or passage, or a path they chose. One man talked about his depth of experience as a caregiver for his lover:

> *If [caregiving] has been a real path . . . It's a strange time for us right now. It's almost a very spiritual time.*

Caregiving may last for only a few months or extend over several years. As in any transition, caregiving demanded time for making meaning of events and experiences as caregivers learned to live and to view their worlds differently. Two partners described the common theme of a life transformed by AIDS caregiving:

> *Joe was diagnosed a little over one year ago and my life has changed forever . . . things keep happening . . . and I have discovered this past year how much work it is.*

> *He was diagnosed in May with a Kaposi's spot. Up until that time AIDS had never entered our relationship. Nobody ever thought about AIDS . . . It's completely changed our lives in a lot of ways. And where we're at right now is . . . we've almost come full circle now. We've worked out a lot of things this past year, dealing with the disease.*

The transition of AIDS caregiving was characterized by both numerous crises and quiescent periods between crises. Common precipitators of crises were usually associated with sudden changes in the PWA's health such as *Pneumocystis* pneumonia, falls, delirium, and acute panic attacks. One caregiver described his frightening experience of finding his lover at home critically ill:

> *I called him at his apartment and he was very, very sick and he was in a lot of denial. And the reality of it was that he was developing cryptococcal meningitis. He was becoming demented and totally out of it . . . He kept dropping the phone and not picking it up. I'd scream into the phone and there'd be no answer . . . finally I said, "I think we've got to go into the hospital." I went to pick him up and he had difficulty buzzing me into the apartment. When I got into the apartment it was a total mess. There was rotting food all over. He didn't know who he was.*

The quiescent times between crises were often viewed by caregivers as "good times." Often during these periods caregivers were able to focus more on their own lives, to create a more peaceful existence, and to increase involvement in community and social activities. One lover, who had experienced many crises with the PWA in the past year, now felt a respite from the difficulties and was enjoying a new sense of well-being:

> *It sounds hard to believe after all these things I've been telling you, but I'm very happy with the way my life is going right now. I have the most wonderful balance in the world, of working at the bakery part-time and being able to live in a very bohemian lifestyle, working in my garden, spending what time I can with Jeff. I am at definitely the most content place in my life than I've been in many, many, many years. I don't think I would do anything different right now.*

Managing and Being Managed by the Illness

This subcategory is defined as vigilantly monitoring the mercurial illness of HIV/AIDS and constantly responding to the relentless demands and uncertainties associated with caregiving tasks. The stages and strategies involved in *Managing and Being Managed* include (a) watching and analyzing, (b) doing for,[2] and (c) coordinating help.

Although present in all categories, uncertainty was most dramatic in *Managing and Being Managed* and reflected the recent appearance of AIDS as a new and poorly understood disease. This uncertainty for caregivers was related to questioning how the disease would unfold, monitoring the symptoms, determining the meaning of symptoms and illness behavior, deciding about treatment options, evaluating the effectiveness of caregiving strategies, and developing confidence in their ability to care for the PWA.

A common example of uncertainty related to monitoring the illness was the attempt to determine the meaning of the PWA's symptoms. This process was evident in the dilemma called, "Is it him or the disease?" Caregivers often questioned the PWA's behavior by asking, "Is this an emotional response to the disease (e.g. depression) or is this just him?" The uncertainty manifest in this question prompted caregivers to be cautious so that they would not overlook important symptoms. Consequently, they seriously questioned whether each symptom indicated a new manifestation of the disease, such as a brain lesion, the beginning of an opportunistic infection, or a milestone suggesting a slow, steady deterioration. In the absence of a physiological explanation, caregivers attempted to resolve the uncertainty by attrib-

---

[2]The language and conceptualization of *Doing For* was influenced by Dr. Kristen Swanson's theoretical development of caring published in *Nursing Research* (Vol. 40, No. 3).

uting symptoms to the PWA's personality. This form of uncertainty was often very stressful, as expressed by one woman caring for her friend:

> *His decision-making skills and abilities could be really impaired and it's important to keep a scope on that in your heads ... It's like, he's crazy now! You know, it's hard to tell, because like I said, he's a pretty far out there person anyway. It's like, "Do you think he's crazy now? What do you guys think? I don't know ... Maybe." ... I mean, he goes out and buys a $300 funeral outfit. Is this crazy behavior?*

Being Managed by the Illness resulted from the relentless nature of caregiving activities and seriousness of the PWA's immune system compromised by HIV infection. Despite the numerous activities involved in managing the illness, the feeling of "never being able to do enough" contributed to the perception of being managed. One mother described how the vigilance of monitoring the disease and the uncertainty of the PWA's behavior translated into the feeling of "24 hours a day on call":

> *You can't leave him alone too long because you never know how the mind's going to be. You never know things. Like one time I went to sleep and I thought he was in his room and he had checked himself back into the hospital.*

For many caregivers, this constant vigilance became a major contributor to the experience of *Being Managed by the Illness*. Overall, the cumulative stresses associated with *Being Managed by the Illness* sometimes resulted in caregiver burnout that seriously affected the individual's quality of life.

Living with Loss and Dying

This subcategory is defined as the process of revising one's plans for living in the world based on the possible or probable death of a loved one. Stages and strategies include: (a) Facing loss, (b) Putting the future on hold, and (c) Maximizing the present.

Three major sources of uncertainty within *Living with Loss and Dying* were described by caregivers: whether to remain hopeful about the PWA's survival, not knowing which illness or opportunistic infection would herald the PWA's death, or not knowing when the death would occur. These uncertainties related to facing loss were very painful for caregivers to contemplate. Yet, death was so commonplace in those with AIDS, and the threat of death so powerful, that most caregivers were unable to deny the reality of a probable death. One man described the uncertainty of his partner's survival during an acute illness:

> *The doctor said, "You know I don't know..." Well, actually when Matt first went into the hospital he was so sick the doctor said, "I don't know if he'll live through the evening or he'll*

*live for..." As the doctor told me, "He might die tonight, he
might die in six months." That was the time for him given.
And I thought, "Well, hmmm, this is an interesting situation."*

Another man wondered how the dying process of his lover would unfold:

*Sometimes I wonder "Will he, you know, will his immune
system just sort of fall apart, and will he have multiple oppor-
tunists and die fairly quickly, within a matter of a few
months, or will there be a prolonged time of morbidity, lots of
time in the hospital, lots of time in which he feels bad and
needs emotional support from me and dies?"*

Both the long-range and short-term future were constant sources of uncertainty for caregivers. Even plans for the most immediate future—tomorrow, this
weekend—were always uncertain because they were contingent on the PWA's
strength and symptomology. Living "one day at a time" became an anchor in the
lives of many caregivers as they struggled with an uncertain future and focused on
the present.

Renegotiating the Relationship

This subcategory is defined as the ongoing process of revising the rules and expectations and striving to reach acceptable balances. Stages and strategies include (a)
Modifying give and take, (b) Coping with dependency, and (c) Minimizing conflict.
Uncertainty within *Renegotiating the Relationship* focused on questioning one's
commitment to caregiving, the rules and expectations of the relationship given the
PWA's illness, and appropriate strategies for interpersonal conflict with someone
who may die soon.

At the outset of illness or the diagnosis of AIDS, caregivers often faced the
fundamental question: "Am I willing to do this?" However, many caregivers did not
recall consciously choosing to become a caregiver, and instead naturally assumed
the role given the nature of their relationship with the PWA. For some caregivers,
the increasing strains and demands associated with caregiving provoked uncertainty
about staying in or leaving the relationship. Despite his initial commitment to caregiving, one 24-year-old man questioned whether he could continue caring for his
lover and cope with the constant changes in their relationship brought about by
AIDS:

*Like any other relationship, you have your ups and
downs, and sometimes there's more downs than ups ... maybe
it's better for us to ... you have to decide whether it's healthier
to be in a relationship or healthier to not be in a relationship
... I've wanted to end the relationship a number of times, but
then again, I say to myself, take some time, you're overreact-*

ing, and say maybe he is doing this because he's dealing with the whole bit and you have to look at it from that respect.

Going Public

This category is defined as managing social relationships and choosing social identification based on information about oneself that is both private and very important. Stages and strategies include (a) Living with secrecy, (b) Asserting oneself, and (c) Balancing risks and benefits. The private and important information focused on the caregiver's involvement with the PWA, and, consequently, his or her association with AIDS. The intent of living with secrecy about one's caregiver status was to protect oneself and the PWA from negative judgements, rejection, ridicule, and discriminatory acts. Because these consequences could be devastating, caregivers had a vested interest in anticipating others' responses and in planning accordingly.

The uncertainty of *Going Public* involved the inability to predict others' reactions to the knowledge that the caregiver was taking care of a person with AIDS. One mother felt apprehensive about responding to commonplace inquiries from friends and acquaintances:

> *I really do have a child who is involved in homosexuality, perhaps, and that is not socially acceptable yet. How do I deal with this? ... My daughter brought this out just last week, and I haven't resolved this issue yet. What am I going to do when I meet a former neighbor or somebody in a grocery store who asks, "How are the kids?"*

Because of their inability to predict the reactions of others, caregivers often orchestrated disclosure by carefully choosing who to tell, by making concrete plans for disclosure, and by staging the type and amount of information given. One woman spent a considerable amount of time with her friend developing a plan about how together they would inform his family:

> *His mother had a lot of problems with homosexuality and with his having AIDS. The day before we started telling his family we had structured a whole process of how he would inform the family, who he would tell first. [We would] sort of gain acceptance on the most promising ground and move through a process. And we had this in place, a plan...*

Containing the Spread of HIV

This subcategory is defined as the fear surrounding the spread of HIV infection and the strategies used to prevent transmission to self and others. Stages and strategies include (a) Confronting fear and personal vulnerability and (b) Doing things differently. Uncertainty about transmission was particularly troubling in the beginning of caregiving. One priest caring for a close friend in a congregate living setting described the initial questions of the group about *Containing the Spread* in response to the PWA's move into the house:

> *What do we do with this kind of thing? What does it mean that he's in the public areas of our house? All the fears of AIDS. What does a person with AIDS have to watch out for in terms of hygiene and all those kinds of things? We had a meeting in which everyone [living in the house] sat down and talked to each other about it.*

Furthermore, some caregivers lacked confidence in the efficacy of preventive measures and were not always reassured by scientific information alone. One wife caring for her husband expressed her mistrust of "safer sex," and had great difficulty resuming their sexual relationship:

> *I know that when I tried to have sex with him I was very fearful. Even though there was protection and everybody told me I was 98% safe, I had fear mixed with a lack of trust, and the whole situation was a great conflict for me.*

One lesbian who was caring for her former lover emphasized the particular uncertainty associated with female-to-female transmission:

> *I used to always wear gloves during sex and now I don't wear them sometimes. And the rubber dams, just forget it. I go on an intuitive basis pretty much. I really make sure I don't have any cuts on me. I'm a total guinea pig. Nobody knows how women are going to transfer it.*

For many partners and spouses, an essential component of confronting fear and vulnerability was facing their own HIV status. Many worried about their own HIV exposure, and uncertainty resurfaced each time they sought periodic AIDS testing. One gay partner described the conflict associated with regular HIV testing:

> *It was funny because I got the results of my latest HIV test, and the next day I flew out of Seattle [on business]. And I'm thinking, God, what if this is positive? But it wasn't, thank God ... And then, once I got the results of the first test back you feel like, I'll live forever. But that doesn't mean a year down the road you won't be. "Oh, no, I thought I was going to escape..."*

▌ DISCUSSION

Chick and Meleis (1986) identified illness, recovery, and loss (all of which are integral to the AIDS family caregiving phenomenon) as precipitators of transitions. According to Murphy (1990, p. 1), "A transitions perspective is valuable because, to the extent that transitions are anticipatory, preparation for role change and prevention of negative effects can be instituted." Although most authors equate transitions with change, work by Golan (1981) supports the interrelationship between transitions and uncertainty found in this study; she defined transitions as "a period of moving from one state of certainty to another, with an interval of uncertainty and change in between" (p. 12).

Uncertainty has been studied primarily in relation to experiences with chronic or life-threatening illnesses (Mishel, 1988; Mishel & Braden, 1987; Mishel & Braden, 1988; Cohen, 1989), and more recently pregnancy (Sorenson, 1990), breast cancer (Hilton, 1988), and AIDS (Gordon & Shontz, 1990; Weitz, 1989). In a hermeneutical inquiry that examined living with the AIDS virus, Gordon and Shontz (1990) identified uncertainty as a major theme which was closely woven into the other themes of feeling infected and infectious, facing death and dying, secrecy, and ambivalence. Weitz (1989) found that uncertainty in the lives of PWAs focused on the acquisition of AIDS, the meaning of symptoms, short-term functioning, living with dignity, and the prognosis of AIDS. Given the uncertainty experienced by PWAs, it is not surprising that similar concerns regarding uncertainty were prevalent among family members in this study.

While uncertainty has been noted in other caregiving situations, such as cancer, it is a relatively unexplored theme in the family caregiving literature. Research about caregiver uncertainty suggests (a) an association between uncertainty and caregiver health (Stetz, 1989), (b) uncertainty related to the course of therapy and outcomes resulted in significant caregiver needs (Blank, Clark, Longman, & Atwood, 1989), (c) uncertainty associated with managing the illness and monitoring symptoms was a significant source of stress for parents of chronically ill children (Cohen, 1989), and (d) the early stages of caregiving for the cognitively impaired elderly were marked with uncertainty and unpredictability (Wilson, 1989). Much of the uncertainty in the family caregiving literature was associated with the illness itself, whereas data in the present study revealed that uncertainty in AIDS caregiving also pertained to loss and dying, interpersonal relationships, contagion, and the presentation of self. Furthermore, uncertainty was an important concern for caregivers, similar to the uncertainty reported by family members of cancer patients (Chekryn, 1985; Germino, 1984).

The results advance understanding of AIDS caregiving uncertainty by integrating a theoretical perspective on transitions, by delineating cultural and social contextual features, and by specifying content areas (that is, according to the five caregiving subcategories). Therefore, the findings highlight directions for developing clinical therapeutics in the areas of AIDS family caregiving and uncertainty. Anticipatory guidance could be an important strategy to help caregivers cope with uncertainty because they can identify it, expect it, accept it, and define which of the uncertain circumstances are appropriate and desirable to change. Anticipating caregiving as a transitional period marked by major changes and a new perspective on what is important in life may help reduce the strain associated with the demands of caregiving. In considering clinical therapeutics for AIDS family caregivers, significant gaps remain in understanding the content and timing of the most appropriate interventions. Longitudinal research designs are best suited to address these gaps because of the transitional nature of caregiving as it changes over time. Longitudinal data about AIDS family caregiving are essential to refine the content and timing of interventions, to maximize therapeutic value, and to enhance cost-effectiveness.

REFERENCES

Baumgarten, M. (1989). The health of a person giving care to the demented elderly: A critical review of literature. *Journal of Clinical Epidemiology, 42,* 1137–1148.

Blank, J. J., Clark, L., Longman, A. J., & Atwood, J. R. (1989). Perceived home care needs of cancer patients and their caregivers. *Cancer Nursing, 12*(2), 78–84.

Blumer, H. (1969). *Symbolic interactionism: Perspective and method.* Englewood Cliffs, NJ: Prentice Hall.

Bowers, B. (1987). Intergenerational caregiving: Adult caregivers and their aging parents. *Advances in Nursing Science, 9*(2), 20–31.

Chekryn, J. (1984). Cancer recurrence: Personal meaning, communication and marital adjustment. *Cancer Nursing, 7,* 491–498.

Chenoweth, B., & Spencer, B. (1986). Dementia: The experience of family caregivers. *The Gerontologist, 26,* 267–272.

Chick, N., & Meleis, A. I. (1986). Transitions: A nursing concern. In P. L. Chinn (Ed.), *Nursing research methodology* (pp. 237–257). Rockville, MD: Aspen.

Cohen, M. H. (1989). The sources and management of uncertainty in life-threatening chronic illness [Abstract]. *Communicating Nursing Research, 22,* 155.

DSHS & Seattle-King County Health Department. (1991). *Washington St/Seattle-King County HIV/AIDS Epidemiology Report,* 1st quarter, p. 1.

Edwards, B. (1988). Stories from the front: How to cope when your lover has ARC or AIDS. In T. Eidson (Ed.), *The AIDS caregiver's handbook* (pp. 206–216). New York: St. Martin's Press.

Ekberg, J., Griffith, N., & Foxall, M. J. (1986). Spouse burnout syndrome. *Journal of Advanced Nursing, 1,* 161–165.

Germino, B. B. (1984). *Family members' concerns after cancer diagnosis.* Unpublished doctoral dissertation, University of Washington, Seattle.

Glaser, B., & Strauss, A. (1967). *The discovery of grounded theory: Strategies for qualitative research.* Chicago: Aldine.

Golan, N. (1981). *Passing through transitions.* New York: Free Press.

Gordon, J., & Shontz, F. (1990). Living with the AIDS virus: A representative case. *Journal of Counseling and Development, 68,* 287–292.

Haque, R. (1989). A family's experience with AIDS. In J. H. Flaskerud (Ed.), *AIDS/HIV Infection: A reference guide for nursing professionals* (pp. 230–240). Philadelphia: W. B. Saunders.

Hepburn, K. (1990). Informal caregivers: Front-line workers in the chronic care of AIDS patients. In *Community based care for persons with AIDS: Developing a research agenda* (pp. 37–42), (DHHS Publication No. (PHS) 90-3456). Washington, DC: U.S. Government Printing Office.

Hilton, B. A. (1988). The phenomenon of uncertainty in women with breast cancer. *Issues in Mental Health Nursing, 9,* 217–238.

Lincoln, Y. S., & Guba, E. G. (1985). *Naturalistic inquiry.* Beverly Hills, CA: Sage.

Livingston, M. (1985). Families who care. *British Medical Journal, 291,* 919–920.

Miller, B., & Montgomery, A. (1990). Family caregivers and limitations in social activities. *Research on Aging, 12,* 72–93.

Mishel, M. (1990). Reconceptualization of the Uncertainty in Illness theory. *IMAGE: Journal of Nursing Scholarship, 22,* 256–262.

Mishel, M. (1988). Uncertainty in illness. *Image, 20,* 225–232.

Mishel, M., & Braden, C. (1987). Uncertainty: A mediator between support and adjustment. *Western Journal of Nursing Research, 9,* 43–57.

Mishel, M., & Braden, M. (1988). Finding meaning: Antecedents of uncertainty in illness. *Nursing Research, 37,* 98–103.

Moffatt, B. C. (1986). *When someone you love has AIDS.* New York: NAL Penguin.

Monette, P. (1988). *Borrowed time.* New York: Avon Books.

Montgomery, R., Gonyea, J., & Hooyman, N. (1985). Caregiving and the experience of subjective and objective burden. *Family Relations, 34,* 19–26.

Murphy, S. A. (1990). Human responses to transitions: A holistic nursing perspective. *Holistic Nursing Practice, 4*(3), 1–7.

Ostrow, D., & Gayle, T. (1986). Psychosocial and ethical issues of AIDS health care programs. *Quarterly Review Bulletin, 12,* 284–294.

Parkes, C. M. (1971). Psycho-social transitions: A field for study. *Social Science & Medicine, 5,* 101–115.

Rabins, P. V., Mace, N. L., & Lucas, M. J. (1982). The impact of dementia on the family. *Journal of the American Medical Association, 248,* 333–335.

Rabins, P. V., Fitting, M. D., Eastham, J., & Fetting, J. (1990). The emotional impact of caring for the chronically ill. *Psychosomatics, 31,* 331–336.

Raveis, V., & Siegel, K. (1990). Impact of caregiving on informal or familial caregivers. In *Community-based care of persons with AIDS: Developing a research agenda* (pp. 17–28). (DHHS Publication Number (PHS) 90-3456). Washington, DC: U.S. Printing Office.

Sandelowski, M. (1986). The problem of rigor in qualitative research. *Advances in Nursing Science, 8*(3), 27–37.

Schoen, K. (1986). Psychosocial aspects of hospice care for AIDS patients. *The American Journal of Hospice Care, 3*(2), 32–34.

Shilts, R. (1987). *And the band played on: Politics, people, and the AIDS epidemic.* New York: St. Martin's Press.

Snyder, B., & Keefe, K. (1985). The unmet needs of family caregivers for frail and disabled adults. *Social Work in Health Care, 10*(3), 1–14.

Sorenson, D. (1990). Uncertainty in pregnancy. NAACOG's *Clinical Issues in Perinatal and Women's Health Nursing, 1,* 289–296.

Stetz, K. (1989). The relationship among background characteristics, purpose in life, and caregiving demands on perceived health of spouse caregivers. *Scholarly Inquiry for Nursing Practice, 3,* 133–159.

Strauss, A. L. (1987). *Qualitative analysis for social scientists.* Cambridge: Cambridge University Press.

Thomas, R. (1987). Family adaptation to a child with a chronic condition. In M. H. Rose & R.

B. Thomas (Eds.). *Children with chronic conditions* (pp. 29–54). New York: Harcourt Brace Jovanovich.

Weitz, R. (1989). Uncertainty and the lives of persons with AIDS. *Journal of Health and Social Behavior, 30,* 270–281.

Wilson, H. S. (1989). Family caregiving for a relative with Alzheimer's dementia: Coping with negative choices. *Nursing Research, 38,* 94–98.

Wolcott, D. L., Fawzy, F. I., & Landsverk, J., & McCombs, M. (1986). AIDS patients' needs of psychosocial services and their use of community service organizations. *Journal of Psychosocial Oncology, 4,* 135–146.

Zarit, S. H., Todd, P. A., & Zarit, J. M. (1986). Subjective burden of husbands and wives as caregivers. A longitudinal study. *The Gerontologist, 26,* 260–266.

Notes

Notes

Notes

Notes

Notes

Notes

Notes

Notes